THE DIET FOR STRONG BONES

Supplements and Diet for Stronger Bones

Robert Galbraith

Copyright

Table of content

Introduction

Once upon a time, in a quaint little town nestled amidst rolling hills and lush forests, lived a young woman named Emma. She was known for her adventurous spirit and love for exploring the natural wonders that surrounded her home. However, there was one thing that dampened her enthusiasm – a persistent and debilitating bone issue that had plagued her since childhood.

Emma had endured years of pain and discomfort due to weak and brittle bones. She had consulted numerous doctors and tried various treatments, but none seemed to provide lasting relief. As the years went by, her condition worsened, and the once-vibrant girl found herself confined to her home, unable to pursue her beloved outdoor adventures.

One day, while aimlessly browsing through the shelves of the town's small library, Emma came across an old and weathered book titled **"The diet for strong bones."** Curiosity piqued, she pulled the dusty volume from the shelf and began to flip through its pages. The book was filled with stories of miraculous recoveries and healing, each tale more incredible than the last.

Among the stories, one particular chapter caught Emma's eye - **"Understanding Bone Health ."** Intrigued, she read on, discovering the story of a person who had suffered from severe bone issues but had miraculously healed through the power of positive thinking, faith, and self-belief. The person in the story had immersed themselves in the written words, treating each sentence like a healing mantra, and slowly, their bones regained strength and vitality.

Inspired by the account, Emma decided to give it a try. She began to read **"The diet for strong bones"** every day, absorbing its words with unwavering faith. With each page turned, she envisioned her bones growing stronger and healthier, free from the limitations that had held her captive for so long.

As days turned into weeks and weeks into months, Emma's determination never wavered. She found solace and hope in the words of the book, and as she read, a newfound sense of peace enveloped her. Slowly but steadily, she noticed changes within herself. Her pain began to subside, and she could move more freely than she had in years.

The townspeople noticed the transformation in Emma, and whispers of her miraculous healing spread like wildfire. Many were skeptical, dismissing it as mere coincidence, but others saw the sparkle return to her eyes and believed in the magic of her journey.

One day, Emma decided to visit her old doctor, the same one who had seen her struggle for so long. As she walked into the clinic, the doctor couldn't believe his eyes. The girl who had once needed crutches to walk now stood tall and strong, radiating an aura of newfound vitality.

Astounded by the transformation, the doctor asked Emma about her healing journey. With a smile on her face, she shared the tale of **"The diet for strong bones"** and how reading its words had breathed life back into her bones. The doctor, though skeptical, could not deny the tangible results before him.

Word of Emma's healing spread far beyond the town, capturing the attention of medical experts and scholars. Some dismissed it as a mere placebo effect, while others were open to exploring the potential of the mind-body connection in healing.

Emma's story became an inspiration to many, and **"The diet for strong bones"** found its way into the hands of countless individuals seeking hope and solace. Whether it was the power of belief or a miraculous coincidence, no one could say for certain. But for Emma, it didn't matter; what mattered was that she had discovered a path to healing, and her bones were now stronger than they had ever been before.

Chapter 1: Importance of Bone Health

Bone health is a crucial aspect of overall well-being that is often overlooked until problems arise. Bones serve as the structural framework of our bodies, providing support, protection, and mobility. They also play a fundamental role in maintaining mineral balance, producing blood cells, and protecting vital organs. Therefore, it is essential to understand and prioritize bone health throughout our lives.

1. Strong Foundation: Just as a solid foundation is vital for a stable building, strong bones form the basis for a healthy body. During childhood and adolescence, bone mass increases rapidly, reaching its peak around the age of 30. Afterward, bone density gradually starts to decline. By building strong bones during youth through a balanced diet and weight-bearing activities, individuals can reduce the risk of bone-related issues later in life.

2. Prevention of Osteoporosis: Osteoporosis is a condition characterized by low bone density and deteriorating bone structure, making bones fragile and prone to fractures. This disease often affects older adults, especially women after menopause. By maintaining optimal bone health through proper nutrition and regular exercise, the risk of developing osteoporosis can be significantly reduced.

3. Reduction of Fracture Risks: Strong and healthy bones are more resilient and less likely to break, even when subjected to external forces. Whether it's a minor fall or a significant impact, individuals with good bone health have a lower risk of fractures and can recover more quickly if an injury does occur.

4. Improved Mobility: Healthy bones enable better mobility and flexibility, allowing individuals to maintain an active lifestyle as they age. This is crucial for maintaining independence and overall quality of life. On the other hand, weak bones can lead to limited mobility, loss of independence, and increased risk of falls.

5. Support for Muscles and Joints: Bones work in conjunction with muscles and joints to facilitate movement. Strong bones provide a solid foundation for muscles to anchor, reducing the strain on joints and preventing joint-related issues such as arthritis.

6. Calcium and Vitamin D Metabolism: Bone health is closely linked to calcium and vitamin D metabolism. Calcium is a key mineral that plays a vital role in bone structure, while vitamin D is necessary for the absorption of calcium from the diet. Insufficient levels of either nutrient can lead to weakened bones and related health problems.

7. Cardiovascular Health: Recent research has suggested a link between bone health and cardiovascular health. Some studies have shown that individuals with osteoporosis might be at a higher risk of heart disease and vice versa. Taking care of bone health could, therefore, have positive effects on cardiovascular health as well.

8. Lifestyle Impact: Several lifestyle factors can affect bone health. Smoking, excessive alcohol consumption, sedentary habits, and poor nutrition can all contribute to decreased bone density and increased risk of fractures.

9. Prevention Through Lifelong Habits: The good news is that bone health can be improved and maintained throughout life. Engaging in weight-bearing exercises, consuming a balanced diet rich in calcium and vitamin D, avoiding smoking and excessive alcohol, and getting regular medical check-ups can all contribute to better bone health.

bone health is a critical aspect of overall health and well-being. Strong and healthy bones provide the foundation for an active and independent life, while poor bone health can lead to various issues, including osteoporosis and an increased risk of fractures. By prioritizing bone health through proper nutrition, exercise, and healthy lifestyle choices, individuals can enjoy the benefits of strong bones and reduce the likelihood of bone-related problems as they age.

The Role of Diet and Supplements

Maintaining strong and healthy bones is essential for overall well-being and quality of life. As we age, bone health becomes increasingly important to prevent conditions like osteoporosis and fractures. While genetics and physical activity play significant roles in bone strength, diet and supplements also play a crucial role in supporting and improving bone health.

1. Calcium:

Calcium is a fundamental mineral for bone health. It provides the structural framework for bones and is essential for their strength. Dairy products like milk, yogurt, and cheese are rich sources of calcium. However, for those who are lactose intolerant or have dietary restrictions, calcium can also be obtained from fortified plant-based milk, leafy greens (such as kale and broccoli), canned fish (with bones), and fortified breakfast cereals.

2. Vitamin D:

Vitamin D is a vital nutrient that aids in the absorption of calcium from the digestive tract and its deposition into bones. The body can produce vitamin D when the skin is exposed to sunlight, but it can also be obtained from dietary sources such as fatty fish (salmon, mackerel, and tuna), egg yolks, and fortified foods. For individuals who have limited sun exposure, vitamin D supplements may be recommended by healthcare professionals.

3. Magnesium:

Magnesium is another mineral that contributes to bone health. It helps convert vitamin D into its active form, facilitating calcium absorption. Nuts, seeds, whole grains, and leafy vegetables are excellent sources of magnesium.

4. Vitamin K:

Vitamin K is necessary for synthesizing proteins involved in bone mineralization. Green leafy vegetables like spinach, kale, and Swiss chard are rich sources of vitamin K. It is worth noting that vitamin K interacts with blood-thinning medications like warfarin, so individuals on such medications should consult their healthcare provider before increasing their vitamin K intake.

5. Protein:

Protein is a crucial component of bone tissue and aids in bone maintenance and repair. A diet with an adequate amount of protein from sources like lean meats, poultry, fish, beans, lentils, and dairy products can positively impact bone health.

6. Omega-3 Fatty Acids:

Omega-3 fatty acids, found in abundance in fatty fish (salmon, sardines, and trout) and flaxseeds, possess anti-inflammatory properties that can support bone health.

7. Phosphorus:

Phosphorus works alongside calcium to maintain bone mineral density. It is found in a wide variety of foods, including dairy products, nuts, seeds, and whole grains.

While a well-balanced diet can provide most of the nutrients necessary for strong bones, some individuals may benefit from supplements, especially if they have specific dietary restrictions or medical conditions that affect nutrient absorption. However, it is essential to consult with a healthcare professional before starting any supplement regimen to ensure appropriate dosages and to avoid any potential interactions with medications.

In addition to diet and supplements, weight-bearing exercises like walking, jogging, dancing, and resistance training are essential for maintaining bone density and strength. A combination of a bone-friendly diet, regular physical activity, and a healthy lifestyle can significantly contribute to optimal bone health and reduce the risk of fractures and bone-related conditions in the long run.

Chapter 2: Understanding Bone Health

Bone health is a crucial aspect of overall well-being and plays a fundamental role in maintaining our mobility, strength, and overall quality of life. Bones provide support to the body, protect vital organs, and act as a reservoir for minerals like calcium and phosphorus. Understanding bone health is essential to prevent conditions such as osteoporosis, fractures, and other skeletal disorders.

1. Bone Structure and Composition:

Bones are complex structures made up of various components. The outer layer, known as cortical bone, is dense and provides strength, while the inner part, called trabecular bone or cancellous bone, has a spongy appearance and supports bone marrow. Bone tissue is a living matrix of cells, collagen fibers, and minerals like calcium and phosphorus. This combination gives bones both flexibility and strength.

2. Factors Affecting Bone Health:

Several factors influence bone health throughout life. Genetics, age, sex, and ethnicity play a significant role in determining bone density and susceptibility to bone diseases. Additionally, lifestyle factors such as diet, physical activity, and exposure to certain substances (like tobacco and alcohol) can impact bone health. Hormones, particularly estrogen and testosterone, are essential in maintaining bone density, which is why menopause in women and age-related hormone changes in men can affect bone health.

3. Peak Bone Mass and Bone Loss:

During childhood and adolescence, the body undergoes rapid bone growth and accumulates what is known as peak bone mass, which occurs around the age of 30. Achieving optimal peak bone mass is crucial as it determines the starting point for bone health as an individual ages. After reaching peak bone mass, bone density gradually declines with age, making bones more susceptible to fractures and osteoporosis.

4. Osteoporosis:

Osteoporosis is a common bone disease characterized by low bone mass and deterioration of bone tissue, leading to increased bone fragility and a higher risk of fractures. Women are more prone to osteoporosis, especially after menopause when estrogen levels decline. Prevention and early detection are essential to managing osteoporosis effectively.

5. Maintaining Bone Health:

To promote and maintain good bone health, several practices should be adopted:

a. Balanced Diet: A diet rich in calcium, vitamin D, and other essential nutrients is crucial for bone health. Dairy products, leafy greens, nuts, and fortified foods are excellent sources of calcium and vitamin D.

b. Physical Activity: Weight-bearing exercises, such as walking, jogging, dancing, and resistance training, help stimulate bone remodeling and strengthen bones.

c. Avoiding Unhealthy Habits: Smoking and excessive alcohol consumption can weaken bones and should be avoided.

d. Bone Density Testing: Regular bone density tests are recommended, especially for postmenopausal women and older adults, to detect bone loss early.

e. Hormone Replacement Therapy: In some cases, hormone replacement therapy may be prescribed to help maintain bone density, particularly for women experiencing menopause.

6. Bone Health Across the Lifespan:
Bone health is a lifelong concern. Building strong bones during childhood and adolescence can help minimize the risk of bone-related problems later in life. As individuals age, it becomes even more

crucial to take proactive steps to maintain bone health.

understanding bone health is vital for maintaining a healthy and active lifestyle throughout life. By adopting healthy habits, getting regular exercise, and following a balanced diet, we can optimize bone health and reduce the risk of bone-related disorders such as osteoporosis. Consulting with healthcare professionals and staying informed about the latest advancements in bone health can also help in the prevention and management of bone-related issues.

Bone Structure and Function

Understanding bone health is crucial for maintaining overall well-being and preventing various skeletal conditions. Bones are the fundamental building blocks of the human body, providing support, protection, and facilitating movement. To comprehend bone health, it is essential to delve into bone structure and function.

Bone Structure:

Bones are complex and dynamic structures composed of a combination of minerals, collagen, and cells. The primary minerals found in bones are calcium and phosphate, which give them their strength and rigidity. Collagen, on the other hand, provides flexibility and resilience to withstand stress. These elements work in harmony to create a durable yet flexible framework.

Bones are categorized into two main types: compact bone and spongy (cancellous) bone. Compact bone forms the outer layer of most bones and is dense and solid, providing strength and protection. Within compact bone, there are numerous small channels called Haversian canals, through which blood vessels and nerves pass, nourishing the bone and maintaining communication with the rest of the body.

Spongy bone, as the name suggests, has a more porous and lattice-like structure. It is found at the ends of long bones and inside vertebrae. The spaces in spongy bone contain bone marrow, which is responsible for producing blood cells and storing fat.

Bone Function:

Bones serve several essential functions in the human body:

1. Support and Protection: Bones provide the framework that supports and maintains the shape of the body. They also protect vital organs, such as the brain (protected by the skull) and the heart and lungs (protected by the ribcage).

2. Movement: Bones, along with muscles, facilitate movement. When muscles contract, they pull on bones, allowing us to perform various activities like walking, running, and even fine motor skills like writing.

3. Mineral Storage: Bones act as a reservoir for essential minerals, particularly calcium and phosphate. These minerals are released into the bloodstream as needed for various bodily functions, such as nerve transmission and muscle contraction.

4. Blood Cell Formation: Bone marrow, located in the cavities of certain bones, is responsible for producing red blood cells, white blood cells, and platelets. This process is called hematopoiesis and is critical for the body's immune function and oxygen transport.

Maintaining Bone Health:

Maintaining strong and healthy bones is vital for overall well-being, especially as we age. Several factors contribute to bone health, including:

1. Calcium and Vitamin D: Adequate calcium intake is essential for building and maintaining bone density. Vitamin D is crucial for the absorption of calcium from the diet. Good dietary sources of calcium include dairy products, leafy greens, and fortified foods.

2. Regular Exercise: Weight-bearing exercises such as walking, running, dancing, and resistance training help stimulate bone growth and strengthen bones.

3. Balanced Diet: A well-balanced diet with sufficient nutrients, including vitamin K, magnesium, and phosphorus, supports bone health.

4. Avoiding Smoking and Excessive Alcohol: Smoking and excessive alcohol consumption can negatively impact bone health and increase the risk of osteoporosis.

5. Bone Density Tests: Regular bone density tests are recommended, especially for individuals at higher risk of osteoporosis, to monitor bone health and detect any potential issues early.

Bone health is essential for maintaining a healthy and active lifestyle. Understanding the structure and function of bones can help us appreciate their significance and make informed decisions to keep them strong and resilient throughout life. By adopting a bone-friendly lifestyle and seeking medical advice when necessary, we can minimize the risk of bone-related issues and improve overall quality of life.

Factors Affecting Bone Health

Understanding bone health is essential for maintaining strong and resilient skeletal structures throughout life. Several factors influence bone health, ranging from lifestyle choices to genetic predisposition. By comprehending these factors, individuals can take proactive measures to promote optimal bone health and reduce the risk of bone-related conditions. Here are some of the key factors affecting bone health:

1. Nutrition:

A balanced and nutrient-rich diet is crucial for maintaining healthy bones. Calcium, phosphorus, and vitamin D are especially important for bone health. Calcium provides the structural framework for bones, phosphorus helps form a mineral matrix, and vitamin D aids in the absorption of calcium. Other nutrients like magnesium, vitamin K, and vitamin C also play supportive roles in bone health. A diet that includes dairy products, leafy greens, nuts, seeds, and fortified foods can contribute to better bone health.

2. Physical Activity:

Regular weight-bearing exercises, such as walking, running, dancing, and resistance training, stimulate bone remodeling and help maintain bone density. Weight-bearing activities put stress on the bones, prompting them to become stronger. Additionally, muscle-strengthening exercises improve balance and coordination, reducing the risk of falls and fractures.

3. Hormonal Balance:

Hormones play a significant role in bone health. Estrogen and testosterone, in particular, help regulate bone density. Women experience a decline in estrogen levels during menopause, leading to accelerated bone loss and an increased risk of osteoporosis. Likewise, low testosterone levels in men can negatively affect bone health. Maintaining hormonal balance through lifestyle choices and, if necessary, hormone therapy can support bone health.

4. Age:

Bone density tends to decrease with age. Peak bone mass is typically reached in early adulthood, around the age of 30, after which bone resorption may exceed bone formation. This natural process of bone loss can be slowed down through proper nutrition, exercise, and other bone-friendly practices.

5. Genetics:

Family history and genetics can influence bone health. Some individuals may have a genetic predisposition to conditions like osteoporosis or certain bone disorders. Understanding one's family medical history can help identify potential risks and encourage proactive measures to maintain bone health.

6. Lifestyle Choices:

Certain lifestyle choices can negatively impact bone health. Smoking and excessive alcohol consumption, for example, can lead to decreased bone density and increase the risk of fractures. Smoking interferes with the body's ability to absorb calcium, while excessive alcohol can interfere with bone formation and nutrient absorption.

7. Medical Conditions and Medications:

Certain medical conditions, like celiac disease, inflammatory bowel disease, and hormonal disorders, can affect nutrient absorption and bone health. Some medications, such as long-term use of corticosteroids, can also weaken bones. Managing underlying medical conditions and being mindful of potential side effects of medications can help preserve bone health.

8. Body Weight:

Maintaining a healthy body weight is essential for bone health. Both being underweight and obese can have negative effects on bones. Underweight individuals may have lower bone density, while obesity can increase the load on bones and lead to excessive wear and tear.

Bone health is influenced by a combination of factors, many of which are within an individual's control. Adopting a well-balanced diet, engaging in regular physical activity, avoiding harmful habits, and managing medical conditions can all contribute to maintaining strong and healthy bones. By being proactive about bone health, individuals can reduce the risk of bone-related conditions and enjoy better overall well-being as they age.

Bone Health and Aging

Understanding bone health becomes increasingly important as we age, as bone-related changes are a natural part of the aging process. As we grow older, our bones undergo various transformations, which can impact their strength, density, and overall health. Being aware of these age-related changes and taking proactive steps to maintain bone health can help minimize the risk of fractures and bone-related conditions. Here's a closer look at bone health and aging:

1. Bone Density Changes:

Bone density tends to peak around the age of 30 and gradually declines thereafter. This decline in bone density is more pronounced in women, especially during and after menopause when estrogen levels decrease significantly. Estrogen plays a critical role in maintaining bone density, and its decline can lead to accelerated bone loss. In men, testosterone levels also decrease with age, contributing to bone density changes.

2. Bone Remodeling:

Throughout life, bones undergo a process called remodeling, wherein old bone tissue is replaced by new bone tissue. In younger individuals, bone formation usually outpaces bone resorption, resulting in overall bone mass gain. However, as we age, this balance may shift, and bone resorption may exceed bone formation, leading to decreased bone mass and density.

3. Increased Risk of Osteoporosis:

Osteoporosis is a condition characterized by weakened and fragile bones, increasing the risk of fractures. Aging is a significant risk factor for osteoporosis due to the decline in bone density and changes in bone architecture. Postmenopausal women and older men are particularly vulnerable to osteoporosis.

4. Fracture Risk:

As bone density decreases, the risk of fractures, especially in the hips, spine, and wrists, increases. Even minor falls or accidents can result in severe fractures, impacting an individual's mobility and quality of life.

5. Muscle Strength and Balance:

Aging is also associated with a gradual loss of muscle mass and strength, which can affect balance and increase the risk of falls. The combination of decreased bone density and muscle weakness can make older adults more susceptible to fractures.

6. Nutritional Considerations:
Maintaining a balanced diet with sufficient nutrients becomes even more critical as we age. Calcium and vitamin D are essential for bone health and can help offset age-related bone loss. However, aging may also bring challenges to nutrient absorption, so it is crucial to pay attention to dietary choices and consider supplements if needed.

7. Exercise for Bone Health:
Regular physical activity, including weight-bearing exercises and muscle-strengthening activities, is vital for preserving bone health in older adults. Weight-bearing exercises, such as walking, jogging, and dancing, help stimulate bone formation, while strength training supports muscle health and improves balance.

8. Preventive Measures:

Taking preventive measures to protect bone health is crucial, especially for older adults. This may include regular bone density tests to monitor bone health, lifestyle modifications to reduce the risk of falls, and discussions with healthcare providers about medications or supplements that can support bone health.

Bone health and aging are closely interconnected. As we age, our bones naturally undergo changes that can impact their density and strength. However, being proactive about bone health through a combination of proper nutrition, regular exercise, and preventive measures can help maintain strong and healthy bones, reducing the risk of fractures and osteoporosis. It's never too late to start taking care of bone health, and with the right approach, older adults can lead active and fulfilling lives with a reduced risk of bone-related issues.

Chapter 3: Essential Nutrients for Strong Bones

Strong and healthy bones are essential for maintaining an active and fulfilling lifestyle. Throughout our lives, our bones continuously remodel, grow, and regenerate. However, as we age, the process of bone loss can outpace bone formation, leading to conditions like osteoporosis and an increased risk of fractures. To maintain optimal bone health, it is crucial to focus on a well-balanced diet that provides the necessary nutrients for strong bones. In this article, we will explore the essential nutrients that play a vital role in maintaining bone health and preventing bone-related issues.

1. Calcium:

Calcium is one of the primary minerals responsible for building and maintaining bone strength. It is the key component of hydroxyapatite, a mineral complex that gives bones their hardness and structure. Adequate calcium intake is vital during childhood and adolescence when bone growth is at its peak, but it remains crucial throughout adulthood and into old age to counteract bone loss.

Good sources of calcium include dairy products such as milk, yogurt, and cheese. For individuals who are lactose intolerant or prefer non-dairy options, fortified plant-based milks, leafy green vegetables like kale and broccoli, and certain nuts and seeds are also excellent sources of calcium.

2. Vitamin D:

Vitamin D is essential for the proper absorption of calcium in the body. Without sufficient vitamin D, even if calcium intake is high, the body may struggle to utilize it effectively, leading to weakened bones. Vitamin D is unique as our bodies can produce it through exposure to sunlight. However, many people may still be deficient in this vitamin due to factors like limited sun exposure, geographical location, or age-related changes in skin's ability to synthesize vitamin D.

Fatty fish (such as salmon and mackerel), fortified dairy products, egg yolks, and cod liver oil are some dietary sources of vitamin D. Additionally, supplements may be recommended for individuals with inadequate sun exposure or those at higher risk of deficiency.

3. Phosphorus:

Phosphorus is another crucial mineral that forms part of the bone's mineral structure, working alongside calcium. It aids in the formation and maintenance of strong bones and teeth. Most people get enough phosphorus through their regular diet, as it is present in a wide range of foods, including meat, fish, poultry, dairy products, nuts, and legumes.

4. Magnesium:

Magnesium is involved in numerous biochemical processes in the body, including those related to bone health. It helps convert vitamin D into its active form, supporting calcium absorption and utilization. Furthermore, magnesium aids in the proper functioning of osteoblasts (cells responsible for bone formation) and helps regulate parathyroid hormone, which plays a role in calcium balance.

Magnesium can be found in foods such as leafy green vegetables, nuts, seeds, whole grains, and legumes.

5. Vitamin K:

Vitamin K is essential for bone health as it regulates the incorporation of calcium into bones, making them stronger and less susceptible to fractures. There are two primary forms of vitamin K: K1 (found in leafy green vegetables like spinach and kale) and K2 (found in fermented foods and certain animal products).

Incorporating these essential nutrients into your daily diet is fundamental for building and maintaining strong bones throughout your life. A well-balanced intake of calcium, vitamin D, phosphorus, magnesium, and vitamin K, in combination with regular weight-bearing exercises, can significantly contribute to optimal bone health and reduce the risk of bone-related issues like osteoporosis. Always consult with a healthcare professional before making significant changes to your diet or taking supplements, especially if you have any underlying health conditions. Remember, strong bones are the foundation for an active and vibrant life at any age.

Calcium: The Building Block of Bones

When it comes to maintaining strong and healthy bones, few nutrients are as crucial as calcium. Calcium is often referred to as the "building block of bones" because it forms the foundation of bone structure and provides the necessary strength to support our bodies. This essential mineral plays a vital role in various physiological processes, from enabling muscle contractions to supporting nerve function. However, its primary function lies in creating and maintaining the structural integrity of our skeletal system. In this article, we will delve deeper into the importance of calcium for bone health and explore the best dietary sources to ensure you meet your daily calcium needs.

The Role of Calcium in Bone Health:

Calcium is a mineral that is continuously being deposited and withdrawn from bones in a process known as "bone remodeling." During childhood and adolescence, when bones are growing rapidly, more calcium is deposited than withdrawn, leading to increased bone density. This process continues until around the age of 30 when peak bone mass is achieved. After that, bone formation and breakdown are in a state of equilibrium.

As we age, especially beyond 50, bone resorption (breakdown) can outpace bone formation, resulting in reduced bone density and increased risk of fractures. This is why ensuring an adequate intake of calcium throughout life is essential to maintain bone health and prevent conditions like osteoporosis.

Calcium Absorption and Vitamin D:

While calcium intake is crucial, it is equally important to focus on factors that influence its absorption. Vitamin D, in particular, plays a pivotal role in calcium absorption. Without sufficient vitamin D, the body cannot efficiently absorb calcium from the digestive system, rendering the mineral less effective.

Vitamin D can be obtained through exposure to sunlight, but dietary sources like fatty fish (salmon, mackerel), fortified dairy products, egg yolks, and certain fortified foods are also important contributors. Combining calcium-rich foods with adequate vitamin D sources enhances calcium absorption and maximizes its bone-strengthening benefits.

Calcium-Rich Foods:

1. Dairy Products: Milk, yogurt, and cheese are well-known sources of calcium. Opt for low-fat or non-fat options if you are mindful of calorie and saturated fat intake.

2. Leafy Greens: Dark, leafy greens like kale, broccoli, bok choy, and collard greens contain significant amounts of calcium. These options are also excellent choices for individuals who follow a plant-based diet.

3. Nuts and Seeds: Almonds, chia seeds, and sesame seeds are calcium-rich additions to your diet. Enjoy them as snacks, sprinkle them on salads, or blend them into smoothies.

4. Fortified Foods: Some breakfast cereals, orange juice, and plant-based milk alternatives are fortified with calcium and vitamin D, making them convenient options for meeting your nutrient needs.

Calcium is undeniably the cornerstone of bone health, providing the strength and structure necessary to support our bodies throughout life. From childhood to old age, ensuring an adequate intake of calcium, in combination with sufficient vitamin D, is vital for maintaining optimal bone density and reducing the risk of fractures and bone-related issues. Embrace a balanced diet that incorporates calcium-rich foods like dairy products, leafy greens, nuts, and seeds, and don't forget to soak up some sunlight or include vitamin D-rich foods to optimize calcium absorption. By taking care of your bones today, you can build a foundation of strength and vitality that will support you for years to come.

Vitamin D: Facilitating Calcium Absorption

Strong and healthy bones are vital for maintaining an active and independent lifestyle. As the foundation of our body's framework, bones provide support, protect organs, and enable movement.

Ensuring the proper intake of essential nutrients is crucial for maintaining bone health throughout life. One such vital nutrient is Vitamin D, which plays a pivotal role in facilitating the absorption of calcium, a mineral essential for building and maintaining strong bones. In this article, we will explore the importance of Vitamin D in bone health and how it enables the absorption of calcium.

The Role of Calcium in Bone Health:

Calcium is an essential mineral that makes up the primary component of bones. It is crucial for maintaining bone density and strength. Not only does calcium support the formation of a sturdy skeleton during childhood and adolescence, but it also plays a key role in preventing bone loss and osteoporosis later in life. Without adequate calcium intake, bones can become weak and brittle, making individuals more susceptible to fractures and injuries.

Vitamin D: The Sunshine Vitamin:

Vitamin D, often referred to as the "sunshine vitamin," is a fat-soluble vitamin that can be synthesized by the body when the skin is exposed to sunlight. It can also be obtained through certain foods and supplements. Vitamin D is essential for various bodily functions, but its most crucial role lies in supporting bone health.

Facilitating Calcium Absorption:

Vitamin D enhances calcium absorption in the small intestine, allowing the body to utilize calcium effectively from dietary sources. Without sufficient levels of Vitamin D, the body struggles to absorb the calcium consumed through foods, even if the diet is rich in calcium-rich items. Consequently, this can lead to a calcium deficiency, weakening bones over time and increasing the risk of fractures.

In addition to promoting calcium absorption, Vitamin D regulates calcium levels in the blood. When calcium intake is inadequate, Vitamin D works to maintain the necessary levels by releasing calcium from the bones. However, this process is not ideal for bone health in the long term, as excessive calcium release weakens bones and contributes to osteoporosis.

Sources of Vitamin D:

1. Sunlight: The most natural and abundant source of Vitamin D comes from exposure to sunlight. When the skin is exposed to sunlight, it synthesizes Vitamin D3, which is then converted into its active form by the liver and kidneys.

2. Foods: While it may be challenging to obtain sufficient Vitamin D from diet alone, certain foods can contribute to Vitamin D intake. Foods rich in Vitamin D include fatty fish (salmon, mackerel, and tuna), fortified dairy products (milk, yogurt, and cheese), egg yolks, and fortified cereals.

3. Supplements: In cases where sun exposure and dietary intake are inadequate, Vitamin D supplements may be recommended by healthcare professionals to ensure optimal levels for bone health.

Vitamin D is a crucial nutrient for maintaining strong and healthy bones throughout life. By facilitating calcium absorption in the body, Vitamin D ensures that bones receive the necessary building blocks for optimal density and strength. Combining a diet rich in calcium with adequate Vitamin D intake, whether through sunlight exposure, foods, or supplements, is essential for preventing bone-related disorders and promoting overall bone health. Always consult with a healthcare professional to determine your specific Vitamin D needs and to develop a personalized plan to support your bone health.

Magnesium: Enhancing Bone Density

Essential Nutrients for Strong Bones: Magnesium - Enhancing Bone Density

In the pursuit of overall well-being, few things are as crucial as maintaining strong and healthy bones. Our skeletal system serves as the structural framework for the body, supporting movement, protecting organs, and ensuring stability. To achieve and sustain strong bones, a combination of essential nutrients is required, and one mineral that often takes the spotlight is magnesium. Magnesium plays a vital role in enhancing bone density and promoting overall bone health. In this article, we will explore the importance of magnesium and its impact on bone density.

The Role of Magnesium in Bone Health:

Magnesium is an essential mineral that participates in numerous biochemical processes throughout the body. While it is often associated with its role in energy production and muscle function, magnesium is equally critical for maintaining healthy bones. About 60% of the body's magnesium resides in the bones, where it helps regulate the balance between bone formation and resorption.

Bone remodeling is a constant process that involves the breakdown of old bone tissue (resorption) and the subsequent formation of new bone tissue. This continuous renewal is essential for maintaining bone strength and preventing fractures. Magnesium plays a crucial role in supporting this delicate balance between bone resorption and formation, contributing to the overall density and integrity of bones.

Enhancing Bone Density:

One of the primary ways magnesium enhances bone health is by influencing bone mineralization. Magnesium is a cofactor for various enzymes involved in the production of osteoblasts, the cells responsible for bone formation. Osteoblasts require an adequate supply of magnesium to synthesize collagen, a crucial protein that forms the matrix for bone mineralization.

Furthermore, magnesium aids in the activation of Vitamin D, another essential nutrient for bone health. As mentioned in previous articles, Vitamin D facilitates calcium absorption, and magnesium contributes to this process by activating the enzyme responsible for converting Vitamin D into its active form. Consequently, this collaborative effort ensures that the absorbed calcium can be effectively utilized for bone mineralization.

Additionally, magnesium helps regulate parathyroid hormone (PTH), which plays a role in maintaining calcium balance. By controlling PTH levels, magnesium indirectly affects calcium levels in the blood, ultimately influencing bone health.

Sources of Magnesium:

A balanced diet rich in magnesium is essential for supporting bone density and overall health. Magnesium can be found in various food sources, including:

1. **Nuts and Seeds:** Almonds, pumpkin seeds, sunflower seeds, and cashews are excellent sources of magnesium.

2. **Leafy Greens:** Spinach, kale, and Swiss chard are packed with magnesium, along with other essential nutrients.

3. Whole Grains: Whole wheat, quinoa, brown rice, and oats provide significant amounts of magnesium.

4. Legumes: Beans, lentils, and chickpeas are magnesium-rich plant-based options.

5. Fish: Fatty fish such as salmon and mackerel contain magnesium, along with beneficial omega-3 fatty acids.

6. Avocado: This creamy fruit is a tasty source of magnesium.

While calcium and Vitamin D often steal the spotlight in discussions about bone health, the importance of magnesium should not be underestimated. Magnesium plays a crucial role in enhancing bone density and supporting overall bone health. By aiding bone mineralization, activating Vitamin D, and regulating calcium balance, magnesium ensures that bones remain strong and resilient throughout life. Including magnesium-rich foods in your diet and maintaining a balanced lifestyle can help promote optimal bone density and reduce the risk of bone-related conditions, allowing you to enjoy a life full of mobility and vitality. As always, it's essential to consult with a healthcare professional to ensure you meet your individual nutrient needs for maintaining strong and healthy bones.

Vitamin K: Promoting Bone Health

When we think about nutrients essential for bone health, Vitamin K might not be the first one that comes to mind. However, this often-overlooked vitamin plays a critical role in maintaining strong and healthy bones. Vitamin K is a group of fat-soluble vitamins that primarily aid in blood clotting, but it also contributes significantly to bone health. In this article, we will delve into the importance of Vitamin K in promoting bone health and its impact on bone density and strength.

The Role of Vitamin K in Bone Health:

Vitamin K is essential for the production of certain proteins in the body, particularly those involved in blood clotting and calcium regulation. Two main forms of Vitamin K are relevant for bone health: Vitamin K1 (phylloquinone) and Vitamin K2 (menaquinone). Vitamin K1 is primarily obtained from leafy green vegetables, while Vitamin K2 is found in fermented foods and certain animal products.

One of the crucial roles of Vitamin K in bone health is its involvement in the carboxylation of specific proteins, particularly osteocalcin and matrix Gla protein (MGP). Osteocalcin is a protein that helps bind calcium to the bone matrix, promoting mineralization and strengthening bones. Matrix Gla protein, on the other hand, helps prevent the unwanted deposition of calcium in soft tissues, which could be detrimental to bone health.

By supporting the carboxylation of these proteins, Vitamin K ensures that calcium is appropriately directed to the bones, where it is needed for bone formation and mineralization, and away from soft tissues, where it can lead to calcification and contribute to vascular and tissue damage.

Promoting Bone Density and Reducing Fracture Risk:

Studies have shown that adequate Vitamin K intake is associated with improved bone density and a reduced risk of fractures, especially in older adults. Higher levels of circulating undercarboxylated osteocalcin, an indicator of inadequate Vitamin K status, have been linked to lower bone mineral density and an increased risk of hip fractures.

Vitamin K has also been found to work synergistically with other bone-supporting nutrients, such as calcium and Vitamin D. Ensuring a balanced intake of these nutrients can further enhance bone health and reduce the risk of bone-related conditions like osteoporosis.

Sources of Vitamin K:

1. Leafy Green Vegetables: Kale, spinach, collard greens, broccoli, and Brussels sprouts are excellent sources of Vitamin K1.

2. Fermented Foods: Natto, a traditional Japanese dish made from fermented soybeans, is particularly rich in Vitamin K2.

3. Animal Products: Certain animal products, such as cheese, egg yolks, and meat, contain small amounts of Vitamin K2.

4. Vegetable Oils: Soybean oil, canola oil, and olive oil are sources of Vitamin K1.

While Vitamin K may not be as well-known as other bone-supporting nutrients, its role in promoting bone health is undeniable. By facilitating the carboxylation of proteins involved in bone mineralization and calcium regulation, Vitamin K ensures that calcium is appropriately directed to the bones, contributing to their density and strength. Including Vitamin K-rich foods in your diet, such as leafy greens and fermented foods, can be beneficial for maintaining optimal bone health and reducing the risk of fractures, particularly in older adults. As always, it is essential to maintain a balanced diet and consult with a healthcare professional to ensure you meet your individual nutrient needs for strong and healthy bones throughout life.

Other Vital Nutrients for Bones

While calcium, Vitamin D, magnesium, and Vitamin K are essential players in promoting bone health, several other vital nutrients also contribute to maintaining strong and resilient bones. A well-rounded and balanced diet that includes a variety of nutrients is crucial for supporting overall bone health and preventing bone-related conditions. In this article, we will explore some of these additional nutrients that play a significant role in supporting strong bones.

1. Phosphorus:

Phosphorus is the second most abundant mineral in the body, with about 85% found in the bones and teeth. It works in tandem with calcium to form the mineral hydroxyapatite, the primary component of bone tissue. Phosphorus is vital for bone mineralization and supports bone strength and density. Dairy products, meat, fish, poultry, nuts, and whole grains are good dietary sources of phosphorus.

2. Vitamin C:

Vitamin C is an antioxidant that plays a crucial role in collagen synthesis. Collagen is a protein that forms the structural framework for bones, providing flexibility and resilience. Including Vitamin C-rich foods like citrus fruits, strawberries, kiwi, bell peppers, and broccoli in your diet can support collagen production and contribute to strong bones.

3. Vitamin A:

Vitamin A is involved in the regulation of bone cell activity and the maintenance of bone density. It aids in the differentiation of osteoblasts, the cells responsible for bone formation. Sources of Vitamin A include carrots, sweet potatoes, spinach, and liver.

4. Zinc:

Zinc is an essential mineral that supports bone health by contributing to bone formation and mineralization. It is a cofactor for various enzymes involved in bone metabolism. Oysters, beef, poultry, beans, and nuts are good sources of zinc.

5. Vitamin B12:

Vitamin B12 is necessary for the production of red blood cells and DNA synthesis, which indirectly supports bone health. It is found primarily in animal products like meat, fish, eggs, and dairy.

6. Copper:

Copper is a trace mineral that participates in collagen synthesis, assisting in the formation of the bone matrix. It also plays a role in the activity of certain enzymes involved in bone development. Copper can be obtained from nuts, seeds, whole grains, and organ meats.

7. Vitamin E:

Vitamin E is an antioxidant that helps protect bone cells from oxidative damage. While more research is needed to fully understand its role in bone health, Vitamin E-rich foods like almonds, sunflower seeds, and spinach can be beneficial as part of a balanced diet.

In addition to calcium, Vitamin D, magnesium, and Vitamin K, several other nutrients are essential for maintaining strong and healthy bones. A well-rounded diet that includes a variety of nutrient-rich foods can provide the necessary support for bone mineralization, bone density, and overall bone health. Including foods rich in phosphorus, Vitamin C, Vitamin A, zinc, Vitamin B12, copper, and Vitamin E can further enhance bone health and contribute to reducing the risk of bone-related conditions. As always, it is advisable to maintain a balanced diet and seek guidance from a healthcare professional to ensure you meet your individual nutrient needs for optimal bone health throughout life.

Chapter 4:. Dietary Sources of Bone-Strengthening Nutrients

Maintaining strong and healthy bones is crucial for overall well-being and mobility throughout life. As we age, our bones tend to lose density and become more susceptible to fractures and osteoporosis. Fortunately, a balanced diet rich in bone-strengthening nutrients can play a significant role in promoting bone health and reducing the risk of bone-related issues.

Here are some essential nutrients and the dietary sources that can help fortify your bones:

1. Calcium:

Calcium is the most well-known mineral when it comes to bone health. It provides structural strength to bones and helps with muscle contractions and nerve transmission. Dairy products are the most abundant sources of calcium, including milk, yogurt, and cheese. For those who are lactose intolerant or follow a plant-based diet, calcium can be obtained from fortified plant-based milk (such as almond, soy, or oat milk), tofu, leafy green vegetables (like kale, collard greens, and broccoli), and almonds.

2. Vitamin D:

Vitamin D is essential for the absorption of calcium in the body. It helps regulate calcium levels and supports bone mineralization. The primary source of vitamin D is sunlight. Spending some time outdoors, especially during sunny days, allows your skin to produce vitamin D naturally. However, dietary sources include fatty fish (such as salmon, mackerel, and sardines), egg yolks, and fortified foods like orange juice, cereal, and dairy alternatives.

3. Vitamin K:

Vitamin K is vital for bone health as it regulates calcium utilization and promotes bone formation. Green leafy vegetables are excellent sources of vitamin K, including spinach, kale, Swiss chard, and collard greens. Additionally, broccoli, Brussels sprouts, and parsley also contribute to your vitamin K intake.

4. Magnesium:

Magnesium plays a role in converting vitamin D into its active form, which aids in calcium absorption. It also supports the structural development of bones. Good dietary sources of magnesium include nuts (almonds, cashews), seeds (pumpkin seeds, flaxseeds), whole grains (brown rice, quinoa, oats), beans, and dark chocolate.

5. Phosphorus:

Phosphorus works in conjunction with calcium to form the mineral crystals that give bones their strength. It is found in a wide range of foods, with high concentrations in dairy products, fish, poultry, red meat, nuts, and whole grains.

6. Protein:

Adequate protein intake is essential for maintaining bone density and muscle mass. The amino acids in protein help in building and repairing bones. Sources of protein that contribute to bone health include lean meats, poultry, fish, eggs, dairy products, legumes (beans, lentils, chickpeas), and tofu.

7. Zinc:

Zinc is a trace mineral involved in bone mineralization and collagen synthesis. It can be obtained from foods such as oysters, beef, chicken, beans, nuts, and whole grains.

Remember that a balanced diet rich in a variety of nutrients is key to promoting bone health. Moreover, it is essential to limit excessive alcohol consumption, avoid smoking, and engage in regular weight-bearing exercises, as they also contribute significantly to overall bone strength and density. If you have specific concerns about your bone health, consider consulting with a healthcare professional or a registered dietitian for personalized advice.

Calcium-Rich Foods

Calcium is a fundamental mineral for building and maintaining strong bones. It is a vital nutrient that not only supports bone health but also plays a crucial role in various physiological processes, such as muscle function, nerve transmission, and blood clotting. Since our bodies cannot produce calcium on their own, it is essential to obtain an adequate amount through our diet. Here are some calcium-rich foods that can help fortify your bones:

1. Dairy Products:
Dairy foods are well-known for their high calcium content, making them a reliable source of this essential mineral.

- **Milk:** Cow's milk is one of the most common sources of calcium. It's rich in readily absorbable calcium and is often fortified with vitamin D for enhanced absorption.

- **Yogurt:** Greek yogurt and regular yogurt are excellent sources of calcium, and they also provide beneficial probiotics for gut health.

- **Cheese:** Cheese varieties like cheddar, mozzarella, and Swiss contain significant amounts of calcium. However, it's essential to consume them in moderation due to their higher fat content.

2. Leafy Greens:

Various leafy green vegetables are not only packed with vitamins and minerals but are also great sources of calcium.

- **Spinach:** This nutrient-dense green contains a substantial amount of calcium. However, it also contains oxalates, which can hinder calcium absorption, so it's good to balance spinach consumption with other calcium sources.

- **Kale:** Rich in calcium and other bone-supporting nutrients like vitamin K and magnesium, kale is a valuable addition to your diet.

- **Collard Greens:** Another calcium powerhouse among leafy greens, collard greens offer a good dose of this bone-strengthening mineral.

3. Fortified Plant-Based Milk:

For individuals who are lactose intolerant or prefer a plant-based diet, there are several calcium-fortified alternatives available.

- **Almond Milk:** Fortified almond milk is a popular dairy-free choice that provides calcium along with a nutty flavor.

- **Soy Milk:** Soy milk is often fortified with calcium and is a good source of plant-based protein.

- **Oat Milk:** Oat milk, made from oats, is another option that may be fortified with calcium and is naturally lower in fat.

4. Fish:

Certain types of fish with edible bones are excellent natural sources of calcium.

- **Canned Salmon:** Canned salmon with bones contains not only calcium but also omega-3 fatty acids, which are beneficial for heart health.

- **Sardines:** These small fish are an exceptional calcium source and are also rich in vitamin D.

5. Fortified Foods:

Many food products are fortified with calcium to boost their nutritional value.

- **Fortified Orange Juice:** Some brands of orange juice are enriched with calcium and vitamin D.

- **Fortified Cereals:** Certain breakfast cereals are fortified with various vitamins and minerals, including calcium.

6. Tofu:

Tofu, a soy-based protein, is often enriched with calcium during the manufacturing process. It serves as a valuable plant-based calcium source for vegans and vegetarians.

Incorporating these calcium-rich foods into your daily diet can significantly contribute to maintaining strong bones and supporting overall bone health. Remember that alongside calcium, it's crucial to ensure sufficient vitamin D intake, as it aids in the absorption of calcium from the digestive tract into the bloodstream. For personalized dietary advice or if you have specific health concerns, consult with a registered dietitian or healthcare professional.

Vitamin D Sources

Vitamin D is a crucial nutrient for bone health as it aids in the absorption of calcium, which is essential for maintaining strong and healthy bones. Here are some dietary sources of vitamin D:

1. Fatty Fish: Fatty fish like salmon, mackerel, sardines, and trout are excellent sources of vitamin D. Just a small serving of these fish can provide a significant amount of the daily recommended intake.

2. Cod Liver Oil: Cod liver oil is a potent source of vitamin D, and a single tablespoon can often fulfill your daily vitamin D requirements.

3. Fortified Foods: Many foods are fortified with vitamin D to help increase the intake of this nutrient. Common fortified foods include fortified milk, orange juice, breakfast cereals, and plant-based milk alternatives like soy milk.

4. Egg Yolks: Egg yolks contain vitamin D, so incorporating eggs into your diet can contribute to your vitamin D intake.

5. Beef Liver: Beef liver contains vitamin D, as well as other essential nutrients, though it should be consumed in moderation due to its high vitamin A content.

6. Cheese: Some types of cheese, like Swiss cheese and cheddar, contain small amounts of vitamin D.

7. Mushrooms: Some varieties of mushrooms are exposed to ultraviolet (UV) light during cultivation, which increases their vitamin D content. These are labeled as "vitamin D enriched" mushrooms.

8. Sunlight: Although not a dietary source, sunlight is one of the most natural ways for the body to produce vitamin D. When your skin is exposed to sunlight, it synthesizes vitamin D. However, the amount of sunlight needed depends on factors like skin type, geographic location, time of day, and season.

It's worth noting that vitamin D is a fat-soluble vitamin, meaning it is better absorbed when consumed with some dietary fat. Additionally, for some individuals with specific health conditions or those living in regions with limited sunlight, supplementation may be recommended to ensure adequate vitamin D intake. As always, it's essential to consult with a healthcare professional before starting anysupplementation regimen

Vitamin K–Rich Diet Options

Vitamin K is another essential nutrient for bone health, as it plays a critical role in the synthesis of proteins necessary for bone formation and mineralization.

Here are some dietary sources of vitamin K:

1. Leafy Green Vegetables: Dark leafy greens are among the best sources of vitamin K. Examples include kale, spinach, collard greens, Swiss chard, and turnip greens.

2. Broccoli: Broccoli is a cruciferous vegetable that contains a significant amount of vitamin K, along with other beneficial nutrients.

3. Brussels Sprouts: Brussels sprouts are another cruciferous vegetable rich in vitamin K.

4. Cabbage: Cabbage, whether green or red, contains vitamin K and can be a nutritious addition to your diet.

5. Spring Onions (Scallions): Spring onions are a good source of vitamin K and can be used in various dishes for added flavor and nutrition.

6. Parsley: Fresh parsley is not only a flavorful herb but also a source of vitamin K.

7. Natto: Natto is a traditional Japanese dish made from fermented soybeans and is exceptionally rich in vitamin K2, a form of vitamin K that is particularly beneficial for bone health.

8. Sauerkraut: Sauerkraut, fermented cabbage, is another source of vitamin K2.

9. Prunes: Prunes, or dried plums, contain a notable amount of vitamin K and can be a tasty way to support bone health.

10. Soybean Oil: Soybean oil is a good source of vitamin K1, which is the form of vitamin K found in plant-based foods.

Remember that vitamin K is a fat-soluble vitamin, so consuming these vitamin K-rich foods with a healthy source of dietary fat can enhance absorption. Additionally, a well-balanced diet that includes a variety of nutrient-rich foods will not only support bone health but overall health and well-being. If you have specific health concerns or conditions, it's always a good idea to consult with a healthcare professional or a registered dietitian for personalized dietary advice.

Incorporating Nutrient-Rich Foods in Everyday Meals

Incorporating nutrient-rich foods for bone health into your everyday meals can be enjoyable and straightforward. Here are some ideas on how to do it:

1. Start with a Nutrient-Packed Breakfast:

- Add fortified cereal or oatmeal topped with vitamin D enriched milk or plant-based milk alternatives.

- Include some sliced fruits like bananas or berries for added nutrients.

- Sprinkle chia seeds or ground flaxseeds for omega-3 fatty acids, which also support bone health.

2. Build Nourishing Lunches:

- Prepare salads with a mix of dark leafy greens (rich in vitamin K) like spinach, kale, or arugula, and toss in some broccoli or Brussels sprouts.

- Add grilled salmon or canned sardines for a dose of vitamin D and calcium.

- Incorporate chickpeas or kidney beans for protein and additional nutrients.

3. Wholesome Snack Options:

- Munch on a handful of almonds or walnuts, as they contain calcium and magnesium, both important for bone health.

- Snack on carrot or celery sticks with hummus (made from chickpeas) for added nutrients.

4. Create Bone-Boosting Dinners:

- Cook stir-fried vegetables using sesame oil (a source of vitamin K) and tofu (for calcium).

- Enjoy a serving of whole-grain pasta with tomato sauce, which contains vitamin K and can be topped with parmesan cheese (calcium source).

- Grill or bake chicken thighs (with the skin) for a source of vitamin D.

5. Delicious Desserts with Nutrients:

- Make a fruit salad with dried prunes and figs (rich in bone-strengthening nutrients) and top with yogurt for added calcium.

6. Don't Forget Vitamin D from Sunlight:

- Spend some time outdoors to get natural sunlight exposure, which helps your body produce vitamin D.

Remember that balanced nutrition is essential, and incorporating a variety of nutrient-rich foods into your diet will have more benefits for your overall health. Additionally, be mindful of portion sizes and try to avoid excessive intake of processed or sugary foods, as they may hinder nutrient absorption or have a negative impact on bone health.

If you have specific dietary restrictions, health conditions, or concerns, consider consulting with a registered dietitian who can provide personalized advice and meal planning tailored to your needs and goals.

Chapter 5: Supplements for Bone Health

Maintaining strong and healthy bones is essential for overall well-being and mobility throughout our lives. As we age, bone health becomes even more crucial to prevent conditions like osteoporosis and fractures. While a balanced diet and regular exercise are the cornerstones of good bone health, sometimes it's beneficial to incorporate supplements that can provide additional support. In this article, we'll explore some of the key supplements known to promote bone health.

1. Calcium:

Calcium is the most well-known mineral for bone health and is a major component of bone tissue. It helps maintain bone density and strength, and it plays a crucial role in muscle function and nerve transmission as well. While dietary sources of calcium include dairy products, leafy greens, and fortified foods, some individuals may need calcium supplements to meet their daily requirements, especially those who are lactose intolerant or have limited dietary calcium intake.

2. Vitamin D:

Vitamin D is essential for the proper absorption of calcium from the intestines. Without sufficient vitamin D, your body cannot efficiently utilize the calcium you consume. Sunlight is a natural source of vitamin D, but many people don't get enough exposure, especially in certain seasons or regions. Therefore, vitamin D supplements can be beneficial, particularly for individuals with limited sun exposure or certain medical conditions that affect vitamin D absorption.

3. Magnesium:

Magnesium is another mineral that supports bone health. It works synergistically with calcium to maintain bone density and strength. Moreover, it aids in the activation of vitamin D, further enhancing calcium absorption. Magnesium-rich foods include nuts, seeds, whole grains, and leafy greens. If your diet lacks these sources, a magnesium supplement can be considered.

4. Vitamin K:

Vitamin K is involved in the synthesis of proteins that regulate bone mineralization. It helps transport calcium into bones and prevents it from accumulating in soft tissues. There are two main forms of vitamin K: K1 (phylloquinone) found in leafy greens and K2 (menaquinone) found in fermented foods and some animal products. A balanced diet usually provides adequate vitamin K, but supplementation may be helpful, especially for those at risk of bone-related issues.

5. Collagen:

Collagen is the primary protein in bone tissue and contributes to bone structure and resilience. As we age, collagen production decreases, affecting bone health. Collagen supplements are gaining popularity as they may promote bone density and reduce the risk of fractures. Some collagen supplements also contain additional bone-supporting nutrients like calcium and vitamin D.

6. Omega-3 Fatty Acids:

Omega-3 fatty acids have anti-inflammatory properties and may help reduce bone loss. They are commonly found in fatty fish, flaxseeds, and chia seeds. While omega-3 supplements are not specifically marketed for bone health, they can contribute to overall well-being and may indirectly support bone health by reducing inflammation.

It's essential to remember that while supplements can be beneficial, they are not a substitute for a healthy lifestyle. They should complement a balanced diet rich in nutrients and regular weight-bearing exercises like walking, running, or resistance training. Before starting any new supplements, it's advisable to consult with a healthcare professional, especially if you have underlying health conditions or take other medications to avoid potential interactions and ensure personalized recommendations.

taking care of your bone health is a lifelong commitment. By incorporating the right supplements, along with a healthy diet and active lifestyle, you can strengthen your skeletal foundation and enjoy a life of strong, healthy bones.

Understanding Bone Health Supplement

Bone health is a vital aspect of overall well-being, and it plays a crucial role in maintaining mobility and independence as we age. While a balanced diet and regular exercise form the foundation of strong bones, some individuals may benefit from adding supplements to their routine to support and enhance bone health. In this article, we will delve deeper into the world of bone health supplements, understanding their role, types, and considerations.

1. Importance of Bone Health Supplements:

Bone health supplements are formulated to provide essential nutrients that support bone density, strength, and overall skeletal integrity. These supplements aim to address potential deficiencies in crucial vitamins and minerals that are integral to bone health. While some individuals may have specific dietary restrictions, medical conditions, or other factors that hinder the optimal absorption of these nutrients, supplements can bridge the gap and ensure the body receives the necessary support for healthy bones.

2. Common Bone Health Supplements:

a. Calcium: As mentioned earlier, calcium is a primary mineral in bone composition, making it one of the most fundamental nutrients for bone health. Calcium supplements are available in various forms, such as calcium carbonate and calcium citrate, and they are often combined with vitamin D for improved absorption.

b. Vitamin D: Vitamin D plays a vital role in facilitating calcium absorption in the intestines, contributing to bone mineralization. Many people have low levels of vitamin D, especially in areas with limited sunlight exposure. Vitamin D supplements help ensure that the body has an adequate supply for optimal bone health.

c. Magnesium: Magnesium works synergistically with calcium and vitamin D to maintain bone density and strength. It aids in converting vitamin D into its active form and promotes calcium uptake into the bones. Magnesium supplements can be beneficial, especially for those with inadequate dietary intake.

d. Vitamin K: Vitamin K is involved in the regulation of calcium, directing it towards bones and preventing it from accumulating in arteries and soft tissues. Vitamin K supplements, particularly the K2 form, are gaining attention for their potential role in bone health.

e. Collagen: Collagen is a critical protein that provides structure and support to bones, joints, and connective tissues. Collagen supplements, often derived from animal or marine sources, may promote bone health and help preserve bone density.

f. Omega-3 Fatty Acids: While not directly marketed for bone health, omega-3 fatty acids have anti-inflammatory properties that may benefit bone health by reducing bone loss and promoting overall well-being.

3. Considerations and Precautions:

Before incorporating bone health supplements into your daily routine, it's essential to consider the following factors:

a. Consultation: Always consult with a healthcare professional, such as a doctor or registered dietitian, before starting any new supplements. They can assess your individual needs, medical history, and potential interactions with medications.

b. Dosage: Follow the recommended dosage guidelines provided by the supplement manufacturer or as advised by your healthcare professional. Taking excessive amounts of certain nutrients can be harmful.

c. Quality: Choose reputable brands and look for supplements that have been third-party tested for quality and purity.

d. Balanced Diet: Remember that supplements should complement a balanced diet, not replace it. Strive to consume a variety of nutrient-rich foods for overall health.

e. Lifestyle Factors: Engaging in weight-bearing exercises and maintaining a healthy lifestyle are essential for bone health. Supplements are not a substitute for these lifestyle choices but can provide additional support.

Bone health supplements can be valuable tools in promoting and maintaining strong, healthy bones. Understanding the different types of supplements available, their roles, and considering individual needs can help individuals make informed decisions about incorporating these supplements into their bone health regimen. Prioritizing bone health through a comprehensive approach that includes supplements, a balanced diet, and an active lifestyle can contribute to a stronger skeletal foundation and a better quality of life.

When to Consider Supplements

Maintaining strong and healthy bones is essential for a vibrant and active life. While a well-balanced diet and regular exercise are key components of bone health, there are certain situations where considering supplements can provide additional support. Here are some instances when it may be appropriate to think about incorporating bone health supplements into your routine:

1. Inadequate Dietary Intake:

If your diet lacks essential nutrients crucial for bone health, such as calcium, vitamin D, magnesium, or vitamin K, supplements can help fill the gaps. This is particularly relevant for individuals with dietary restrictions, allergies, or those following restrictive eating patterns, which can lead to insufficient intake of bone-supporting nutrients.

2. Age-Related Bone Changes:

As we age, our bodies may become less efficient at absorbing and utilizing nutrients necessary for bone health. Additionally, older individuals might be less physically active, further impacting bone density and strength. In such cases, bone health supplements can be beneficial in supporting aging bones and reducing the risk of osteoporosis and fractures.

3. Limited Sunlight Exposure:

Vitamin D, often referred to as the "sunshine vitamin," is synthesized in the skin in response to sunlight. If you live in regions with limited sunlight, spend little time outdoors, or frequently use sunscreen, you may have lower vitamin D levels. In such instances, vitamin D supplements can help maintain adequate levels for proper calcium absorption and bone health.

4. Medical Conditions or Medications:

Certain medical conditions and medications can affect bone health. For example, gastrointestinal disorders that impair nutrient absorption may lead to deficiencies in essential bone-supporting nutrients. Similarly, certain medications, like glucocorticoids used to manage inflammation, can negatively impact bone density. In such cases, supplements may be recommended by healthcare professionals to support bone health.

5. Menopause and Hormonal Changes:

During menopause, hormonal changes can lead to a decline in estrogen levels, which plays a protective role in bone health. As a result, women approaching or going through menopause may be at an increased risk of bone loss. In consultation with a healthcare provider, menopausal women may consider supplements containing calcium, vitamin D, and other bone-supporting nutrients.

6. Active Lifestyle and Bone Stress:

Individuals who engage in intense physical activities, such as athletes and those with physically demanding occupations, may put additional stress on their bones. In these cases, supplements that support bone repair and maintenance, like collagen and certain minerals, could be considered to aid in recovery and prevent injuries.

7. Family History of Bone Conditions:

If you have a family history of osteoporosis or other bone-related conditions, it's essential to be proactive about bone health. In addition to a balanced diet, bone health supplements can be part of a preventive approach to support your skeletal system.

Before starting any bone health supplements, it's crucial to seek guidance from a qualified healthcare professional. They can assess your individual needs, review your medical history, and determine whether supplements are appropriate for you. Additionally, they can recommend the right type and dosage of supplements tailored to your specific requirements.

Bone health supplements can be valuable additions to your wellness routine when certain factors impact your ability to get all the necessary nutrients through diet alone. By being mindful of your nutritional intake, staying physically active, and seeking professional advice when needed, you can take proactive steps to support and maintain strong, healthy bones throughout your life.

Types of Bone Supplements

Maintaining strong and healthy bones is essential for overall well-being and quality of life. As we age, our bone density tends to decrease, making us more susceptible to fractures and osteoporosis. A balanced diet rich in calcium, vitamin D, and other nutrients is crucial for bone health. However, some individuals may find it challenging to obtain all the necessary nutrients through their diet alone. In such cases, bone supplements can be a valuable addition to their routine. Let's explore some of the common types of bone supplements:

1. Calcium Supplements:
Calcium is a vital mineral that plays a central role in bone health. It provides the structural framework for bones and teeth and helps in maintaining bone

density. When dietary calcium intake is insufficient, calcium supplements can help bridge the gap. Calcium carbonate and calcium citrate are the two most common forms of calcium supplements. They are available in various strengths and often combined with vitamin D for better absorption.

2. Vitamin D Supplements:

Vitamin D is crucial for the proper absorption of calcium from the gastrointestinal tract into the bloodstream. It aids in the formation and maintenance of strong bones. The primary source of vitamin D is sunlight, but certain populations might have limited sun exposure or difficulty absorbing it, making supplementation necessary.

3. Vitamin K Supplements:

Vitamin K is essential for bone health as it assists in the production of proteins that regulate bone metabolism. One such protein is osteocalcin, which helps bind calcium to the bone matrix. Vitamin K2, in particular, has been associated with improved bone mineral density and reduced risk of fractures.

4. Magnesium Supplements:

Magnesium is involved in several biochemical reactions that support bone health. It helps convert vitamin D into its active form, enhances calcium absorption, and plays a role in the synthesis of collagen, a key component of bone structure.

5. Phosphorus Supplements:

Phosphorus is another mineral that contributes to bone health by forming a structural part of the bone mineral matrix. It works in tandem with calcium to provide strength and rigidity to bones.

6. Collagen Supplements:

Collagen is the most abundant protein in the human body and a crucial component of bones, tendons, ligaments, and cartilage. Collagen supplements may support bone health by promoting bone density and reducing the risk of fractures.

7. Strontium Supplements:

Strontium is a trace mineral that has shown potential in supporting bone health by increasing bone formation and reducing bone resorption.

Strontium ranelate, a prescription medication containing strontium, has been used in some cases of osteoporosis.

It is important to note that while supplements can be beneficial for individuals with specific nutrient deficiencies or those at risk of bone-related issues, they should not replace a balanced diet. Moreover, excessive intake of certain supplements may lead to adverse effects. It is always recommended to consult with a healthcare professional or a registered dietitian before starting any new supplement regimen, as they can provide personalized advice based on individual health needs and conditions.

In addition to supplements, engaging in weight-bearing exercises, maintaining a healthy lifestyle, and avoiding habits like smoking and excessive alcohol consumption also contribute significantly to optimal bone health.

Potential Risks and Side Effects

While bone health supplements can be beneficial for individuals with specific nutrient deficiencies or those at risk of bone-related issues, it's essential to be aware of potential risks and side effects associated with their use. Taking supplements without proper guidance or in excessive amounts can lead to adverse effects. Here are some potential risks and side effects of bone health supplements:

1. Calcium Supplements:
Taking too much calcium from supplements may result in hypercalcemia, a condition characterized by high levels of calcium in the blood. Hypercalcemia can lead to symptoms such as constipation, nausea, vomiting, abdominal pain, excessive thirst, and frequent urination. Long-term excessive calcium intake may also contribute to kidney stones in some individuals.

2. Vitamin D Supplements:

While vitamin D is crucial for bone health, excessive intake of vitamin D supplements can lead to vitamin D toxicity or hypervitaminosis D. Symptoms of vitamin D toxicity include nausea, vomiting, poor appetite, weakness, and even kidney problems. Prolonged vitamin D toxicity can cause hypercalcemia and negatively impact bone health.

3. Vitamin K Supplements:

Vitamin K supplements are generally considered safe when taken at recommended dosages. However, excessive amounts of vitamin K supplements may interfere with certain medications, like blood thinners (anticoagulants), and affect blood clotting.

4. Magnesium Supplements:

Magnesium supplements are generally well-tolerated when taken as directed. However, excessive magnesium intake from supplements can lead to diarrhea, nausea, and abdominal cramping. Individuals with kidney problems should be cautious with magnesium supplements, as they may lead to magnesium buildup in the body.

5. Phosphorus Supplements:

Phosphorus supplements are typically unnecessary for individuals with a balanced diet, as phosphorus is readily available in many foods. Excessive phosphorus intake, particularly from supplements, can disrupt the balance of calcium and phosphorus in the body, potentially weakening bones.

6. Collagen Supplements:

Collagen supplements are generally considered safe for most people when taken at recommended dosages. However, some individuals may experience mild digestive issues, such as bloating or heartburn. People with allergies to collagen sources (e.g., fish, shellfish) should avoid collagen supplements derived from those sources.

7. Strontium Supplements:

Strontium supplements, specifically strontium ranelate, have been associated with rare but severe side effects, including cardiovascular events. Due to these risks, strontium ranelate has been discontinued in some countries and is generally not recommended as a first-line treatment for osteoporosis.

It's important to emphasize that supplements should not replace a balanced diet. Obtaining nutrients from natural food sources is the best way to support bone health. Moreover, certain supplements may interact with medications or medical conditions, making it essential to consult with a healthcare professional before adding any new supplements to your routine.

For individuals with specific bone health concerns, a healthcare provider or a registered dietitian can conduct assessments and recommend appropriate supplements based on individual needs and health status. In some cases, a comprehensive bone health evaluation may be necessary to identify the most suitable interventions.

while bone health supplements can be beneficial, it is crucial to use them judiciously, adhere to

recommended dosages, and seek professional
advice when necessary to minimize potential risks
and side effects.

Chapter 6: The Role of Exercise in Building Strong Bones

When it comes to maintaining optimal health, one aspect that often gets overlooked is bone health. Our bones provide the structural framework for our bodies and play a crucial role in protecting our organs, supporting our muscles, and allowing us to move freely. As we age, the density and strength of our bones naturally decline, making us more susceptible to fractures and osteoporosis. However, regular exercise has been proven to be a powerful ally in building and maintaining strong bones throughout life.

1. Stimulating Bone Formation: Engaging in weight-bearing exercises, such as walking, jogging, dancing, and resistance training, puts stress on the bones. This stress stimulates bone-forming cells called osteoblasts, encouraging them to produce new bone tissue. Over time, this process can increase bone density, making the bones stronger and less prone to fractures.

2. Enhancing Bone Mineral Density: Bone mineral density (BMD) refers to the amount of minerals, such as calcium and phosphorus, present in bone tissue. Exercises that load the bones, like weightlifting or jumping, have been shown to increase BMD. Higher BMD means better bone strength and a reduced risk of fractures, especially in postmenopausal women and older adults who are more vulnerable to osteoporosis.

3. Maintaining Bone Mass: As we age, our bodies may naturally lose bone mass, leading to weaker bones. However, regular exercise can help slow down this process. Engaging in both weight-bearing and muscle-strengthening exercises can assist in preserving bone mass, thus mitigating the effects of bone loss that occur with age.

4. Improving Balance and Coordination: Exercise not only strengthens bones but also helps improve balance and coordination. This is particularly important in preventing falls, as strong bones combined with better balance can significantly reduce the likelihood of fractures in the event of a fall.

5. Promoting Hormonal Balance: Hormones play a crucial role in bone health. Exercise can help regulate hormone levels, particularly those related to bone health, such as estrogen and testosterone. This is particularly relevant for postmenopausal women, as decreased estrogen levels can accelerate bone loss.

6. Reducing the Risk of Osteoporosis: Osteoporosis is a condition characterized by low bone density and an increased risk of fractures. Engaging in regular exercise throughout life can significantly reduce the risk of developing osteoporosis, making it a crucial preventive measure against this debilitating condition.

7. Adaptable to All Ages: The benefits of exercise on bone health are not limited to specific age groups. While engaging in physical activity during childhood and adolescence can help build strong bones for the future, incorporating exercise into adulthood and old age can maintain bone strength and reduce the risk of fractures later in life.

It's important to note that the effectiveness of exercise in building strong bones depends on several factors, including the type, intensity, and frequency of the exercises, as well as an individual's overall health and nutritional status. Before starting any exercise regimen, especially for individuals with pre-existing conditions, it's crucial to consult with a healthcare professional or a certified fitness trainer to ensure that the chosen exercises are safe and appropriate for their specific needs.

exercise plays a vital role in building and maintaining strong bones throughout life. From stimulating bone formation to improving balance and reducing the risk of osteoporosis, physical activity offers numerous benefits for bone health. By incorporating regular exercise into our daily routines and adopting a healthy lifestyle, we can give our bones the support they need to keep us strong and mobile for years to come.

Weight-Bearing Exercises

Weight-bearing exercises play a central role in building strong bones and promoting overall bone health. These exercises involve activities that force the bones to support the body's weight against gravity. The stress placed on the bones during weight-bearing exercises triggers a series of physiological responses that lead to increased bone density and strength. Here are some key points about the role of weight-bearing exercises in building strong bones:

1. Types of Weight-Bearing Exercises: Weight-bearing exercises can be classified into two main categories: high-impact and low-impact exercises. High-impact exercises, such as running, jumping, and plyometrics, involve both feet leaving the ground simultaneously and create a greater force on the bones. Low-impact exercises, like brisk walking, stair climbing, and dancing, involve one foot staying on the ground at all times, exerting less force on the bones.

2. Bone Remodeling Process: The stress applied to bones during weight-bearing exercises triggers a process called bone remodeling. This process involves the breakdown of old bone tissue by cells called osteoclasts and the subsequent formation of new bone tissue by osteoblasts. Over time, this continuous remodeling cycle helps to increase bone density and improve bone quality.

3. Building Bone Mass and Strength: Regular participation in weight-bearing exercises stimulates bone cells to lay down more mineral deposits, primarily calcium and phosphorus, resulting in increased bone mass and strength. This is particularly important during childhood and adolescence when bones are still growing and developing.

4. Benefits for Adults and Seniors: Weight-bearing exercises are not only beneficial for children and adolescents; they also play a crucial role in maintaining bone health throughout adulthood and into old age. Engaging in weight-bearing activities helps to slow down age-related bone loss, reducing the risk of osteoporosis and fractures.

5. Impact on Specific Bones: Different weight-bearing exercises can have varying effects on specific bones. For example, exercises that involve the lower body, like walking and running, primarily target the bones of the legs, hips, and lower spine. On the other hand, exercises that engage the upper body, like weightlifting and push-ups, can benefit the bones in the arms, shoulders, and upper spine.

6. Balancing with Muscle-Strengthening Exercises: While weight-bearing exercises are excellent for bone health, a comprehensive exercise routine should also include muscle-strengthening exercises. Strong muscles help to support and protect the bones, reducing the risk of injuries.

7. Safety Considerations: Although weight-bearing exercises offer significant benefits for bone health, it's essential to perform them with proper form and technique to avoid injuries. Beginners or individuals with specific health conditions should start slowly and gradually increase the intensity of their workouts under the guidance of a fitness professional.

8. Lifestyle and Nutrition: While weight-bearing exercises contribute to strong bones, a healthy lifestyle and balanced nutrition are equally crucial. A diet rich in calcium, vitamin D, and other essential nutrients for bone health complements the benefits of exercise.

weight-bearing exercises are a fundamental component of any bone-strengthening exercise regimen. Whether through high-impact activities like running or low-impact exercises like brisk walking, weight-bearing exercises stimulate bone remodeling, increase bone mass, and improve bone strength. By incorporating these exercises into a well-rounded fitness routine and maintaining a healthy lifestyle, individuals can significantly enhance their bone health and reduce the risk of bone-related issues as they age.

Resistance Training for Bone Strength

Resistance training, also known as strength training or weightlifting, is a powerful form of exercise that plays a significant role in building strong bones and promoting overall bone health. Unlike weight-bearing exercises that primarily stress the bones through impact and gravitational forces, resistance training places mechanical stress on the bones through the use of weights or resistance bands. This type of exercise stimulates bone growth, enhances bone density, and complements weight-bearing exercises to create a comprehensive bone-strengthening routine. Here are some key points about the role of resistance training in building strong bones:

1. Mechanical Loading on Bones: Resistance training involves the application of external resistance to muscles, which indirectly applies mechanical stress to the bones. This stress signals the bones to adapt and become stronger to handle the increased load placed on them during the exercises.

2. Promoting Bone Mineral Density: Just like weight-bearing exercises, resistance training stimulates the formation of new bone tissue, leading to increased bone mineral density (BMD). Higher BMD makes the bones more resistant to fractures and reduces the risk of osteoporosis.

3. Targeting Specific Bone Areas: One of the significant advantages of resistance training is its ability to target specific bone areas. Different exercises can focus on particular bones or groups of bones, allowing for a more customized approach to bone strength development.

4. Building Muscle Mass: Resistance training not only benefits bone health but also helps in building and maintaining muscle mass. Strong muscles provide additional support to the bones, reducing the risk of injuries and fractures.

5. Progressive Overload: An essential principle of resistance training is progressive overload. As individuals become stronger, they gradually increase the resistance, challenging their bones and muscles further. This gradual progression is key to continued improvements in bone strength and overall fitness.

6. Safety and Proper Technique: To ensure the effectiveness and safety of resistance training for bone strength, it's crucial to use proper form and technique. Beginners or those new to strength training should seek guidance from a qualified fitness trainer to design a suitable program and learn the correct execution of exercises.

7. Variety of Exercises: Resistance training offers a wide variety of exercises that can be adapted to individual preferences and needs. From free weights like dumbbells and barbells to machines and resistance bands, there are plenty of options to suit different fitness levels and goals.

8. Balancing with Other Exercise Modalities: While resistance training is excellent for building bone strength, it's essential to incorporate other forms of exercise, such as weight-bearing activities and cardiovascular workouts, for overall fitness and bone health.

9. Benefits for All Ages: Resistance training is beneficial for people of all ages. While younger individuals can use it to build peak bone mass, older adults can use it to slow down age-related bone loss and maintain bone strength.

Resistance training is a valuable tool in building strong bones and promoting bone health. By incorporating resistance exercises into a well-rounded fitness routine that includes weight-bearing activities and a balanced diet, individuals can enhance their bone mineral density, improve bone strength, and reduce the risk of fractures and osteoporosis. As with any exercise program, it's essential to start at an appropriate level, progress gradually, and seek professional guidance to ensure safe and effective training.

Balance and Flexibility Exercises

While weight-bearing exercises and resistance training are crucial for building strong bones, balance and flexibility exercises also play a significant role in promoting bone health and reducing the risk of falls and fractures. These exercises focus on improving stability, coordination, and range of motion, all of which contribute to better overall bone health. Here are some key points about the role of balance and flexibility exercises in building strong bones:

1. **Enhancing Stability:** Balance exercises challenge the body to maintain stability and equilibrium, which helps improve proprioception (awareness of body position) and balance control. This, in turn, reduces the risk of falls, especially in

older adults who are more susceptible to fractures due to decreased bone density.

2. Strengthening Supporting Muscles: Balance exercises often engage the smaller stabilizing muscles that are not fully activated during weight-bearing and resistance exercises. These supporting muscles play a crucial role in maintaining proper posture and protecting the bones from injuries.

3. Improving Bone Alignment: Flexibility exercises, such as stretching, help maintain or improve joint flexibility and range of motion. Proper bone alignment and joint function are essential for reducing stress on the bones and preventing injuries.

4. Preventing Fractures: Improved balance and flexibility can significantly reduce the risk of fractures, especially in older adults. Falls are a common cause of fractures in this age group, and by enhancing balance and flexibility, the likelihood of falls can be minimized.

5. Reducing Joint Stress: Flexibility exercises help keep the joints supple and mobile, reducing the stress placed on them during daily activities and exercise. This can be particularly beneficial for individuals with conditions like arthritis, where joint health is critical.

6. Incorporating Variety: Balance and flexibility exercises offer a diverse range of activities, such as yoga, tai chi, Pilates, and various stretches. These exercises can be easily adapted to individual fitness levels and needs.

7. Joint Health and Cartilage Support: Certain flexibility exercises, like yoga, can promote joint health by encouraging synovial fluid circulation and providing nourishment to the cartilage, which cushions the bones at the joints.

8. Mind-Body Connection: Many balance and flexibility exercises involve a strong mind-body connection, encouraging individuals to focus on their movements, breathing, and posture. This mindfulness can lead to improved body awareness and better overall body mechanics.

9. Complementary to Other Exercises: Incorporating balance and flexibility exercises into a comprehensive fitness routine complements the benefits of weight-bearing and resistance training. Together, these exercises provide a well-rounded approach to bone health and overall well-being.

10. Suitable for All Ages: Balance and flexibility exercises are suitable for people of all ages. They can be especially beneficial for older adults as part of a fall prevention strategy, but they are equally valuable for younger individuals to maintain joint health and prevent injuries.

balance and flexibility exercises are essential components of a comprehensive bone-strengthening exercise regimen. These exercises improve stability, joint function, and range of motion, reducing the risk of falls and fractures while promoting overall bone health. By incorporating a variety of balance and flexibility exercises into a well-balanced fitness routine, individuals can enhance their bone strength, improve posture, and enjoy better mobility throughout their lives. As always, consulting with a fitness professional or healthcare provider is recommended, especially for individuals with specific health concerns or mobility limitations.

Chapter 7: Lifestyle Practices for Optimal Bone Health

Maintaining strong and healthy bones is essential for overall well-being and quality of life. As we age, bone health becomes increasingly important as the risk of osteoporosis and fractures rises. Fortunately, there are several lifestyle practices that can promote optimal bone health and help prevent bone-related issues. Incorporating these practices into your daily routine can make a significant difference in the long run:

1. Balanced Diet:

A well-balanced diet rich in essential nutrients is crucial for bone health. Calcium and vitamin D are particularly important. Calcium is the primary building block of bones, while vitamin D helps the body absorb calcium efficiently. Foods high in calcium include dairy products, leafy greens (such as broccoli and kale), fortified cereals, and canned fish with bones (like salmon and sardines). Vitamin D can be obtained from sunlight exposure and dietary sources like fatty fish, egg yolks, and fortified foods.

2. Regular Exercise:

Weight-bearing and resistance exercises play a key role in maintaining bone density and strength. Weight-bearing exercises, like walking, running, dancing, and stair climbing, require your bones to support your body weight, stimulating bone formation. Resistance exercises, such as weightlifting and resistance band workouts, put stress on the bones, leading to increased bone density over time.

3. Avoid Smoking and Limit Alcohol:

Smoking has been linked to decreased bone density and an increased risk of fractures. Similarly, excessive alcohol consumption can interfere with the body's ability to absorb calcium and negatively affect bone health. Limiting or quitting smoking and moderating alcohol intake are vital for supporting strong bones.

4. Get Enough Sleep:

Adequate sleep is essential for bone health as it allows the body to repair and regenerate tissues, including bones. During deep sleep stages, the body releases growth hormones that contribute to bone remodeling and repair. Aim for 7-9 hours of quality sleep each night to promote overall health, including bone health.

5. Maintain a Healthy Weight:

Being either underweight or overweight can impact bone health negatively. Maintaining a healthy weight through a balanced diet and regular exercise helps ensure that bones are not put under excessive strain, reducing the risk of fractures and joint problems.

6. Monitor Calcium Intake:

While calcium is vital for bone health, excessive intake through supplements may lead to kidney stones and other health issues. It's generally best to obtain most of your calcium from food sources and consult with a healthcare professional before taking calcium supplements.

7. Be Cautious with High-Impact Activities:

While exercise is essential for bone health, high-impact activities may increase the risk of injury, especially if you're just starting or have underlying bone issues. Always consult with a fitness expert or healthcare provider before engaging in high-impact exercises.

8. Bone Density Testing:

If you're at an increased risk of osteoporosis or have concerns about your bone health, consider getting a bone density test. This painless and non-invasive test can assess your bone mineral density and identify potential issues early on, allowing for timely intervention and lifestyle adjustments.

Remember that bone health is a lifelong commitment. By adopting these lifestyle practices, you can proactively support your bones and reduce the risk of bone-related problems as you age. As always, consult with a healthcare professional before making significant changes to your lifestyle or if you have specific health concerns.

Quitting Smoking and Limiting Alcohol Intake

1. Quitting Smoking:

Smoking is detrimental to overall health, and it also has a negative impact on bone health. Here's how smoking affects your bones and why quitting is crucial for optimal bone health:

- **Decreased Bone Density:** Smoking has been associated with lower bone density, making bones more prone to fractures and osteoporosis. The harmful chemicals in cigarettes can interfere with the body's ability to absorb calcium, a critical mineral for bone strength.

- **Impaired Bone Healing:** Smoking can impair the healing process of fractures and bone injuries. The toxins in cigarettes restrict blood flow and reduce the delivery of vital nutrients to the bones, leading to slower healing times and potentially complications during the recovery process.

- Increased Risk of Osteoporosis: Studies have shown that long-term smokers, especially women, are at a higher risk of developing osteoporosis, a condition characterized by weak and fragile bones.

- Accelerated Bone Loss: Smoking has been linked to an accelerated rate of bone loss, particularly in postmenopausal women. This can further contribute to the development of osteoporosis and increase the risk of fractures.

2. Limiting Alcohol Intake:

Moderate alcohol consumption may have some health benefits, but excessive or long-term heavy drinking can have adverse effects on bone health. Here's why it's essential to limit alcohol intake for maintaining strong bones:

- **Reduced Bone Formation:** Chronic alcohol consumption interferes with the body's ability to form new bone tissue. This can lead to decreased bone density and an increased risk of fractures.

- **Calcium Imbalance:** Alcohol can disrupt the body's calcium balance, impairing calcium absorption and leading to calcium loss through urine. Over time, this can weaken bones and contribute to osteoporosis.

- **Increased Risk of Falls:** Alcohol impairs coordination and balance, increasing the risk of falls and fractures, especially in older individuals.

- **Liver Function and Bone Health:** Chronic alcohol abuse can negatively impact liver function, affecting the activation of vitamin D, which is necessary for calcium absorption. As a result, this can lead to weakened bones and compromised bone health.

Tips for Quitting Smoking and Limiting Alcohol Intake:

1. Seek Support: Quitting smoking and reducing alcohol consumption can be challenging, so seeking support from friends, family, or support groups can make the process easier.

2. Set Realistic Goals: Gradually reduce your smoking and drinking habits rather than attempting to quit cold turkey. Set achievable goals and celebrate your progress.

3. Find Alternatives: Replace smoking and drinking habits with healthier alternatives. For example, engage in physical activities, pick up a new hobby, or practice relaxation techniques to cope with stress.

4. Identify Triggers: Recognize the triggers that lead you to smoke or drink excessively and find ways to avoid or cope with them differently.

5. Consult with Professionals: If you're finding it challenging to quit smoking or reduce alcohol intake on your own, don't hesitate to seek guidance from healthcare professionals or addiction specialists.

By quitting smoking and limiting alcohol intake, you can significantly improve your bone health and reduce the risk of osteoporosis and fractures. These lifestyle changes, combined with a balanced diet, regular exercise, and other bone-supporting practices, will contribute to maintaining strong and healthy bones throughout your life.

Maintaining a Healthy Weight

Maintaining a healthy weight is essential for overall well-being, and it also plays a crucial role in supporting optimal bone health. Both being underweight and overweight can have adverse effects on bone density and strength. Here's why maintaining a healthy weight is important for your bones and how to achieve it:

1. Impact of Being Underweight on Bone Health:

Being underweight, especially with insufficient body fat, can lead to several issues that negatively impact bone health:

- **Decreased Bone Mass:** Adequate body fat is essential for the production of estrogen, a hormone that helps protect bones. In women, low body weight can lead to hormonal imbalances that result in reduced bone density.

- **Nutritional Deficiencies:** Underweight individuals may not be getting enough essential nutrients, including calcium and vitamin D, which are crucial for bone health.

- **Increased Risk of Osteoporosis:** Low body weight and bone mass are risk factors for osteoporosis, a condition characterized by weak and brittle bones.

2. Impact of Being Overweight on Bone Health:

While excess body weight does provide some extra mechanical stress on bones, obesity can also have detrimental effects on bone health:

- Increased Pressure on Joints: Excess body weight puts additional pressure on joints, leading to wear and tear of the joint surfaces and potentially causing joint pain and discomfort.

- Inflammation: Obesity is associated with chronic inflammation, which can negatively affect bone health and contribute to bone loss over time.

- Vitamin D Storage: Vitamin D is stored in fat tissues, and in overweight individuals, vitamin D may be less available for use in maintaining bone health.

Tips for Achieving and Maintaining a Healthy Weight for Optimal Bone Health:

1. Balanced Diet: Adopt a balanced and nutritious diet that includes a variety of foods rich in calcium, vitamin D, protein, and other essential nutrients.

Choose whole grains, lean proteins, fruits, vegetables, and low-fat dairy products to support bone health and overall well-being.

2. Regular Exercise: Engage in weight-bearing exercises and resistance training to help maintain bone density and promote healthy bones. Weight-bearing exercises include activities where you support your body weight on your feet, such as walking, jogging, dancing, and hiking. Resistance training with weights or resistance bands helps to strengthen muscles, which in turn supports the bones.

3. Portion Control: Be mindful of portion sizes and avoid overeating. Even when consuming healthy foods, excessive calorie intake can lead to weight gain.

4. Stay Hydrated: Drink plenty of water throughout the day. Sometimes, thirst can be mistaken for hunger, leading to unnecessary calorie intake.

5. Avoid Crash Diets: Avoid crash diets or extreme weight loss programs, as they can result in nutrient deficiencies and bone loss. Gradual and sustainable weight loss, if needed, is healthier for both bones and overall health.

6. Seek Professional Guidance: If you have concerns about your weight or need assistance in achieving a healthy weight, consult with a healthcare provider or a registered dietitian. They can provide personalized advice and support to help you reach your goals.

Maintaining a healthy weight is a vital component of promoting optimal bone health. Whether you need to gain or lose weight, making informed and sustainable lifestyle choices can significantly benefit your bones and contribute to a healthier and more active life.

Reducing Bone Health Risks

In addition to adopting positive habits to support bone health, it is equally important to reduce bone health risks that could potentially harm your bones. By being aware of these risks and taking preventive measures, you can further protect your bones and maintain their strength and density. Here are some lifestyle practices to help you reduce bone health risks:

1. Prevent Falls and Fractures:

Falls and fractures can have a significant impact on bone health, especially as we age. Taking steps to prevent falls can help reduce the risk of bone injuries. Some preventive measures include:

- Keep your living space well-lit to improve visibility and reduce tripping hazards.
- Install handrails on stairs and in bathrooms to provide support and stability.

- Use non-slip mats or rugs to prevent slipping on smooth surfaces.
- Wear proper footwear with good traction and support.
- Engage in regular exercise to improve balance and coordination.

2. Avoid Excessive Long-Term Use of Certain Medications:

Some medications, such as certain corticosteroids and anticonvulsants, can negatively impact bone health if used for extended periods. If you are prescribed these medications, discuss potential bone health risks with your healthcare provider. They may recommend periodic bone density tests and advise on strategies to mitigate the impact on bone health.

3. Manage Medical Conditions:

Certain medical conditions can affect bone health, such as hormonal imbalances (e.g., thyroid disorders, diabetes), gastrointestinal disorders (e.g., celiac disease), and rheumatoid arthritis. Proper management of these conditions in consultation with healthcare professionals can help minimize their impact on bone health.

4. Avoid Prolonged Sedentary Behavior:

Prolonged periods of inactivity or sedentary behavior can contribute to bone loss and weaken muscles. Make an effort to incorporate regular physical activity into your daily routine. Weight-bearing exercises, strength training, and flexibility exercises can all contribute to better bone health.

5. Monitor Bone Health with Regular Check-Ups:

If you are at risk for bone-related issues, such as osteoporosis, or if you have a family history of bone problems, consider getting regular bone density tests. Early detection and intervention can help prevent further bone loss and reduce the risk of fractures.

6. Maintain a Healthy Posture:

Poor posture can put undue stress on certain areas of the body, leading to discomfort and an increased risk of fractures. Practice good posture when sitting, standing, and lifting objects to reduce strain on your bones and spine.

7. Avoid Excessive Alcohol Consumption:

As mentioned earlier, excessive alcohol consumption can negatively affect bone health. If you choose to drink, do so in moderation, following recommended guidelines.

8. Do Not Smoke:

Smoking is harmful to bones, as it can lead to decreased bone density and slow down the healing process of bone injuries. Quitting smoking is crucial for maintaining optimal bone health.

By being mindful of these bone health risks and taking proactive steps to reduce them, you can significantly improve the health and strength of your bones. Always consult with healthcare professionals for personalized advice and guidance, especially if you have specific health concerns or risk factors related to bone health.

Chapter 8: Bone Health throughout Life Stages

Bone health is a vital aspect of overall well-being throughout life stages. Our skeletal system provides the framework and support for our bodies, protects internal organs, and allows us to move and perform various activities. Maintaining strong and healthy bones is essential for preventing injuries, promoting mobility, and reducing the risk of bone-related diseases, such as osteoporosis. Let's explore bone health considerations at different life stages:

1. Childhood and Adolescence:

Bone development begins before birth and continues throughout childhood and adolescence. During these stages, bones grow rapidly, and the body lays down a significant amount of bone mass. Adequate nutrition, especially calcium and vitamin D, is critical during these years. Calcium is the primary building block of bones, while vitamin D facilitates its absorption.

Encouraging physical activity is also essential for promoting bone health during childhood and adolescence. Weight-bearing exercises like running, jumping, and playing sports help stimulate bone growth and increase bone density.

2. Early Adulthood:

By early adulthood, typically in the mid-20s, peak bone mass is reached. It's crucial to continue focusing on a balanced diet rich in calcium, vitamin D, and other bone-supporting nutrients. It's worth noting that reaching optimal peak bone mass is essential as it provides a buffer against bone loss that occurs with aging.

Engaging in regular exercise and maintaining an active lifestyle also helps preserve bone density and strength. However, this is also the time when certain lifestyle factors can affect bone health negatively, such as smoking, excessive alcohol consumption, and a sedentary lifestyle.

3. Adulthood:

As individuals progress into adulthood, it becomes essential to maintain the bone mass achieved during early adulthood. Consuming a diet that includes calcium-rich foods like dairy products, leafy greens, and fortified products, along with adequate vitamin D, remains crucial.

Weight-bearing exercises should continue to be a part of one's routine, as well as incorporating strength training exercises. Resistance training helps build and maintain muscle mass, which indirectly supports bone health.

4. Pregnancy and Lactation:

During pregnancy and lactation, a woman's body undergoes significant hormonal changes, which can affect bone health. The developing fetus requires a substantial amount of calcium for bone growth, so it's vital for pregnant women to ensure adequate calcium intake.

Some pregnant women may experience increased calcium absorption from their diet, but for others, supplements may be necessary under medical supervision. After childbirth, if breastfeeding, mothers also need to maintain their own bone health while providing nutrients to their baby.

5. Midlife and Menopause:

As individuals enter their 40s and 50s, bone mass may start to decline gradually. In women, the postmenopausal stage can lead to accelerated bone loss due to reduced estrogen levels, making them more susceptible to osteoporosis.

To mitigate bone loss during midlife and beyond, a well-balanced diet, including calcium and vitamin D, is still crucial. Weight-bearing exercises and strength training remain beneficial, as they help maintain bone density and muscle mass.

6. Older Adults:

In the elderly population, bone health becomes a significant concern due to the increased risk of fractures and osteoporosis. Preventive measures, including a bone-friendly diet, exercise, and falls prevention strategies, become even more critical.

Medical evaluations, including bone density scans, can help assess bone health and identify potential issues early on. Additionally, healthcare providers may prescribe medications or supplements to support bone health in older adults.

bone health is a lifelong commitment that begins in childhood and continues throughout every life stage. Proper nutrition, regular exercise, and healthy lifestyle choices are key factors in maintaining strong and healthy bones, preventing bone-related issues, and promoting overall well-being. It's essential to be proactive about bone health and work closely with healthcare professionals to address any concerns or risk factors as we age.

Bone Health in Childhood and Adolescence

Bone health is a crucial aspect of overall growth and development during childhood and adolescence. These formative years lay the foundation for strong and resilient bones that will support individuals throughout their lives. During this period, bones are still growing and increasing in density, making it essential to provide the necessary nutrients and lifestyle factors to promote optimal bone health. Let's delve into the significance of bone health in childhood and adolescence:

1. Importance of Calcium and Vitamin D:

Calcium and vitamin D play a central role in bone health. Calcium is the primary mineral responsible for bone strength and structure, while vitamin D aids in the absorption of calcium from the digestive system. Together, these nutrients help in the formation of healthy bones and teeth.

During childhood and adolescence, when bones are rapidly growing, it is crucial to ensure an adequate intake of calcium-rich foods. Dairy products like milk, yogurt, and cheese are excellent sources of calcium. Additionally, leafy greens, nuts, seeds, and fortified plant-based milk alternatives are also good options.

Vitamin D is synthesized in the skin when exposed to sunlight, but dietary sources such as fatty fish, egg yolks, and fortified foods can contribute to meeting the recommended intake.

2. Physical Activity and Weight-Bearing Exercises:

Regular physical activity is vital for bone health during childhood and adolescence. Weight-bearing exercises, such as running, jumping, dancing, and team sports, are particularly beneficial as they place stress on the bones, stimulating bone growth and density.

Engaging in physical activity also helps to improve coordination, balance, and muscle strength, reducing the risk of injuries and fractures.

3. Limiting Sedentary Lifestyle:

In the modern digital age, sedentary behaviors, such as prolonged screen time and reduced physical activity, have become more prevalent among children and adolescents. Excessive sedentary behavior can negatively impact bone health and overall well-being.

Encouraging children to limit screen time and engage in physical activities or sports is crucial for maintaining healthy bones and promoting a healthy lifestyle.

4. Healthy Eating Habits:

In addition to calcium and vitamin D, a balanced diet with adequate amounts of other essential nutrients is vital for overall bone health. Nutrients like phosphorus, magnesium, vitamin K, and vitamin C also contribute to bone development and maintenance.

Encouraging a diet rich in fruits, vegetables, whole grains, lean proteins, and healthy fats helps ensure that children and adolescents receive a wide range of nutrients to support their growing bones.

5. Avoiding Harmful Habits:

During this stage of life, it's essential to avoid harmful habits that can negatively impact bone health. For example, excessive consumption of sugary drinks can displace calcium-rich beverages and lead to decreased calcium intake.

Additionally, smoking and excessive alcohol consumption should be strongly discouraged, as they can interfere with bone growth and increase the risk of fractures.

6. Regular Health Check-ups:

Regular visits to healthcare professionals allow for monitoring growth and development, as well as identifying any potential issues with bone health. Addressing concerns early on can help prevent more significant problems in the future.

Bone health in childhood and adolescence forms the basis for a healthy and strong skeletal system throughout life. Adequate intake of calcium and vitamin D, along with regular physical activity and a balanced diet, are essential for supporting optimal bone development during these critical stages. By promoting healthy habits and prioritizing bone health early on, individuals can lay the groundwork for a lifetime of strong and resilient bones.

Bone Health for Young Adults and Middle-Aged Individuals

Bone health continues to be a vital aspect of overall well-being as individuals transition from adolescence to young adulthood and into middle age. During these life stages, maintaining strong and healthy bones remains essential for supporting daily activities, preventing injuries, and reducing the risk of bone-related conditions such as osteoporosis. Let's explore the considerations for bone health in young adults and middle-aged individuals:

1. Young Adults (20s to 30s):
In early adulthood, individuals have reached their peak bone mass, which is the highest level of bone

density achieved during their lifetime. The focus during this stage shifts from bone growth to maintaining the bone mass acquired during adolescence.

- **Nutrition:** While it's essential to continue consuming a balanced diet rich in calcium and vitamin D, young adults should also pay attention to other nutrients that support bone health. Adequate intake of magnesium, phosphorus, vitamin K, and vitamin C is crucial for maintaining bone density.

- **Physical Activity:** Regular exercise remains essential for bone health in young adults. Weight-bearing exercises, resistance training, and activities that promote balance and flexibility help maintain bone density and muscle strength.

- **Lifestyle Factors:** Young adulthood can be a time of increased social activities and sometimes unhealthy habits. It's important to avoid excessive alcohol consumption, which can adversely affect bone health, and refrain from smoking, as it can hinder calcium absorption.

- **Stress Management:** High levels of chronic stress can lead to hormonal imbalances that may affect bone health. Engaging in stress-reducing activities such as yoga, meditation, or spending time in nature can be beneficial.

2. Middle-Aged Individuals (40s to 50s):

As individuals progress into middle age, bone mass may start to decline gradually. For women, the postmenopausal stage can lead to accelerated bone loss due to reduced estrogen levels.

- **Nutrition:** Middle-aged individuals should continue to focus on a bone-friendly diet, ensuring adequate calcium, vitamin D, and other essential nutrients. It may be beneficial to consult with a healthcare provider about the need for supplements if dietary intake is insufficient.

- **Physical Activity:** Regular exercise remains essential in middle age. Weight-bearing exercises and strength training help maintain bone density and reduce the risk of fractures. Additionally, exercises that improve balance and coordination can help prevent falls, which are a significant concern for bone health.

- Bone Density Testing: In middle age, it's a good idea to discuss bone density testing with a healthcare provider. This can help assess bone health and identify any potential issues early on.

- Hormone Levels: For women experiencing menopause, hormone replacement therapy may be an option to consider for preserving bone density. However, this decision should be made in consultation with a healthcare provider, considering individual health needs and risks.

- Healthy Habits: Continuing to avoid harmful habits such as smoking and excessive alcohol consumption is essential for maintaining bone health in middle age.

- Medical Conditions: Middle-aged individuals should be aware of any medical conditions or medications that may impact bone health. Some health conditions and medications can affect bone density, so discussing these concerns with a healthcare provider is crucial.

Bone health remains a priority throughout life, even as individuals transition from young adulthood to middle age. By focusing on a well-balanced diet, regular physical activity, and healthy lifestyle choices, individuals can continue to support their bone health during these critical life stages. It's essential to be proactive about bone health and work closely with healthcare professionals to address any concerns or risk factors as individuals age.

Bone Health Considerations for Seniors

Bone health is a paramount concern during the senior years. As individuals age, their bones naturally undergo changes, becoming more fragile and susceptible to fractures and osteoporosis. However, with proper care, attention, and lifestyle choices, seniors can maintain strong and healthy bones to support their overall well-being and independence. Let's explore the key considerations for bone health in seniors:

1. Nutrition:

Adequate nutrition is vital for maintaining bone health in seniors. As aging affects the body's ability to absorb nutrients, it becomes even more critical to focus on a well-balanced diet. Seniors should ensure they are getting sufficient calcium, vitamin D, vitamin K, and other essential nutrients for bone health.

- **Calcium:** Dairy products, fortified plant-based milk alternatives, leafy greens, and canned fish with bones are excellent sources of calcium.

- **Vitamin D:** Spending time outdoors in the sunlight can help the body produce vitamin D. Dietary sources of vitamin D include fatty fish, egg yolks, and fortified foods.

- **Vitamin K:** Leafy green vegetables like kale, spinach, and broccoli are good sources of vitamin K.

2. Physical Activity:

Regular physical activity is essential for seniors to maintain bone density and muscle strength. Weight-bearing exercises, such as walking, hiking, dancing, and low-impact aerobics, help stimulate bone remodeling and prevent bone loss.

- **Strength Training:** Resistance exercises using free weights, resistance bands, or weight machines can help build and maintain muscle mass, which indirectly supports bone health.

- **Balance and Flexibility:** Activities like tai chi and yoga can improve balance, flexibility, and coordination, reducing the risk of falls and fractures.

3. Fall Prevention:

Falls are a major concern for seniors, as they can lead to severe injuries, especially for individuals with compromised bone health. Taking steps to prevent falls is crucial:

- **Home Safety:** Remove tripping hazards, ensure proper lighting, and install grab bars in bathrooms to create a safe living environment.

- **Regular Vision Checks:** Maintaining good vision is vital for avoiding obstacles and hazards that may lead to falls.

- **Assistive Devices:** Seniors with mobility challenges may benefit from using canes, walkers, or other assistive devices to maintain stability and prevent falls.

4. Medication and Health Management:

Certain medications and health conditions can impact bone health. Seniors should work closely with healthcare providers to manage chronic conditions and medications that may affect bone density.

- **Medication Review:** Regularly reviewing medications with a healthcare provider can identify potential side effects or interactions that may impact bone health.

5. Avoiding Harmful Habits:

Seniors should refrain from smoking and limit alcohol consumption, as these habits can adversely affect bone health.

6. Bone Density Testing:

Doctors may recommend bone density testing (DXA scan) to assess bone health and identify osteoporosis or osteopenia early on. Depending on the results, appropriate measures can be taken to manage bone health effectively.

7. Lifestyle and Social Engagement:

Maintaining an active and engaged lifestyle can positively impact bone health in seniors. Staying socially connected, pursuing hobbies, and participating in community activities can promote mental and emotional well-being, which can indirectly influence physical health, including bone health.

Bone health is a critical consideration for seniors, and implementing a comprehensive approach to maintain strong bones is essential. With proper nutrition, regular physical activity, fall prevention strategies, and appropriate medical management, seniors can optimize their bone health, reduce the risk of fractures, and enhance their overall quality of life in their golden years.

Chapter 9: Common Bone Health Issues and Solutions

Bone health is a crucial aspect of overall well-being, as our bones provide structural support for our bodies and protect vital organs. However, various factors can impact bone health, leading to common bone health issues. Fortunately, many solutions and preventive measures can help maintain strong and healthy bones throughout life.

Common Bone Health Issues:

1. Osteoporosis: Osteoporosis is a prevalent bone disease characterized by low bone mass and deterioration of bone tissue, making bones fragile and susceptible to fractures. It often develops gradually and is more common in older individuals, particularly post-menopausal women. Factors such as a lack of calcium and vitamin D, sedentary lifestyle, smoking, and excessive alcohol consumption contribute to its development.

2. Osteoarthritis: While osteoarthritis primarily affects the joints, it can also have an impact on bone health. This condition involves the breakdown of cartilage, leading to joint pain and stiffness. Over time, the increased stress on bones near affected joints can result in bone damage and loss of bone density.

3. Rheumatoid Arthritis: This autoimmune disorder affects the joints, causing inflammation that can damage bones and lead to bone loss. People with rheumatoid arthritis are at an increased risk of osteoporosis and fractures due to the chronic inflammation in the joints.

4. Fractures: Fractures can occur due to various reasons, such as falls, accidents, or underlying bone conditions like osteoporosis. Fractures, especially in older individuals, can have serious consequences for overall health and mobility.

Solutions and Preventive Measures:

1. A Balanced Diet: Consuming a diet rich in calcium and vitamin D is essential for maintaining bone health. Dairy products, leafy greens, nuts, and fish are excellent sources of these nutrients. Supplements may be necessary, especially for those with dietary restrictions or who have difficulty absorbing nutrients.

2. Regular Exercise: Engaging in weight-bearing exercises, such as walking, jogging, dancing, or strength training, helps build and maintain bone density. Exercise also improves balance and coordination, reducing the risk of falls and fractures.

3. Quit Smoking and Limit Alcohol: Smoking negatively impacts bone health, while excessive alcohol consumption can lead to bone loss. Quitting smoking and moderating alcohol intake can significantly benefit bone health.

4. Fall Prevention: Taking steps to prevent falls is crucial, especially for older individuals who are more susceptible to fractures. Installing handrails, removing tripping hazards, and ensuring proper lighting in living spaces can help reduce the risk of falls.

5. Medical Check-ups: Regular health check-ups, especially for post-menopausal women and older adults, can help detect bone health issues early on. Early diagnosis allows for timely intervention and management.

6. Medication and Treatment: For individuals with diagnosed bone health issues like osteoporosis, medications and treatments prescribed by healthcare professionals can help manage and improve bone density.

7. Lifestyle Modifications: Maintaining a healthy lifestyle overall, including stress management, adequate sleep, and a balanced diet, supports bone health and general well-being.

8. Bone Density Testing: Doctors may recommend bone density testing, such as a DEXA scan, to assess bone health and identify potential issues.

Bone health is a vital aspect of overall health and should not be overlooked. By adopting a proactive approach through a balanced diet, regular exercise, and lifestyle modifications, individuals can reduce the risk of bone health issues and enjoy strong and healthy bones throughout life. For those with existing bone health conditions, seeking medical advice and adhering to prescribed treatments can help manage and improve bone density, reducing the risk of fractures and other complications.

Osteoporosis: Causes, Symptoms, and Prevention

Causes:

Osteoporosis occurs when the body loses too much bone, makes too little bone, or both, leading to weakened and brittle bones. Several factors contribute to the development of osteoporosis:

1. Age: Bone mass peaks in early adulthood and gradually decreases with age. As people get older, bone loss can outpace bone formation, increasing the risk of osteoporosis.

2. Gender: Women are more susceptible to osteoporosis, especially after menopause, due to the decrease in estrogen levels, which plays a protective role in bone density.

3. Hormonal Changes: Imbalances in hormones, such as thyroid hormones, sex hormones, and cortisol, can affect bone health.

4. Family History: A family history of osteoporosis or fractures may increase an individual's risk of developing the condition.

5. Dietary Factors: A diet low in calcium and vitamin D can lead to reduced bone density and increase the risk of osteoporosis.

6. Physical Inactivity: Lack of weight-bearing exercise and a sedentary lifestyle contribute to bone loss.

7. Smoking and Alcohol: Both smoking and excessive alcohol consumption can weaken bones and accelerate bone loss.

8. Certain Medications and Health Conditions: Long-term use of corticosteroids, anticonvulsants, and some other medications, as well as certain health conditions like rheumatoid arthritis, can increase the risk of osteoporosis.

Symptoms:

In the early stages, osteoporosis may not cause any noticeable symptoms. As the condition progresses, common symptoms and signs include:

1. Back Pain: Persistent or sudden back pain may result from fractures or collapsed vertebrae.

2. Loss of Height: Osteoporosis-related fractures in the spine can lead to a gradual loss of height over time.

3. Posture Changes: Individuals with osteoporosis may develop a stooped posture or a hunched back due to fractures in the vertebrae.

4. Fractures: Osteoporotic bones are more susceptible to fractures, particularly in the hips, wrists, and spine. Fractures caused by minimal impact or even without apparent trauma can be a sign of osteoporosis.

Prevention:
Preventing osteoporosis involves adopting healthy lifestyle habits and reducing risk factors. Here are some preventive measures:

1. Dietary Changes: Ensure a balanced diet rich in calcium and vitamin D. Dairy products, leafy greens, nuts, and fortified foods are good sources of these nutrients.

2. Weight-Bearing Exercise: Engage in weight-bearing and muscle-strengthening exercises regularly to promote bone health.

3. Avoid Smoking and Limit Alcohol: Quit smoking, and limit alcohol intake to reduce the risk of bone loss.

4. Hormone Replacement Therapy (HRT): For postmenopausal women, HRT may help maintain bone density. However, it should be discussed with a healthcare professional, as it carries potential risks.

5. Fall Prevention: Take precautions to prevent falls, such as removing hazards at home, using assistive devices, and maintaining proper lighting.

6. Bone Density Testing: Discuss with a doctor if a bone density test is recommended, especially for individuals at higher risk.

7. Medication and Supplements: In some cases, doctors may prescribe medications or supplements to help manage osteoporosis.

8. Regular Health Check-ups: Regularly visit a healthcare professional for check-ups and bone health assessments.

By taking proactive steps to prevent osteoporosis, individuals can maintain strong and healthy bones, reduce the risk of fractures, and enhance overall quality of life, especially as they age. It's essential to work with healthcare professionals to create a personalized prevention plan based on individual risk factors and health status.

Osteopenia: Early Detection and Management

Osteopenia is a condition characterized by lower-than-normal bone density, but it is not as severe as osteoporosis. It is considered a precursor to osteoporosis and, if left untreated, can progress to a more severe bone loss condition. Early detection and proactive management are essential to prevent further bone density loss and reduce the risk of developing osteoporosis. Here's how osteopenia can be detected and managed:

Early Detection:

1. Bone Density Testing: The most effective way to detect osteopenia is through a bone density test, also known as dual-energy X-ray absorptiometry (DEXA) scan. This non-invasive test measures bone mineral density at various sites in the body, typically the spine, hip, and forearm. It provides a T-score, which compares an individual's bone density to that of a healthy young adult of the same sex. A T-score between -1.0 and -2.5 indicates osteopenia.

2. Risk Assessment: Healthcare professionals may conduct a comprehensive risk assessment to identify factors that contribute to bone density loss.

This assessment includes evaluating age, gender, family history, lifestyle factors, and medical history.

Management:

1. Lifestyle Modifications: Adopting healthy lifestyle habits is a key component of managing osteopenia. This includes:

- **Nutrition:** Ensuring an adequate intake of calcium and vitamin D through diet or supplements. Dairy products, leafy greens, fish, and fortified foods are good sources of these nutrients.

- **Weight-Bearing Exercise:** Engaging in weight-bearing and resistance exercises regularly to strengthen bones and improve bone density. Activities like walking, dancing, and weightlifting are beneficial.

- **Avoiding Harmful Habits:** Quitting smoking and limiting alcohol intake to promote bone health.

2. Medications: In some cases, healthcare professionals may recommend medications to slow down bone density loss and reduce the risk of fractures. Bisphosphonates, selective estrogen receptor modulators (SERMs), and other medications may be prescribed based on individual needs and health status.

3. **Hormone Replacement Therapy (HRT):** For post-menopausal women, hormone replacement therapy may be considered, but its benefits and risks should be carefully evaluated with a healthcare professional.

4. **Regular Follow-ups and Monitoring:** It is essential to have regular follow-up appointments with a healthcare provider to monitor bone density and assess the effectiveness of the management plan.

5. **Fall Prevention:** Minimizing the risk of falls is crucial to prevent fractures, especially for individuals with osteopenia, who may have slightly reduced bone density. Measures to prevent falls

include maintaining a clutter-free living space, using assistive devices if necessary, and ensuring proper lighting.

6. Educate and Empower: Understanding osteopenia, its progression to osteoporosis, and the importance of adherence to the management plan can empower individuals to take charge of their bone health.

Early detection and proactive management of osteopenia can significantly slow down bone density loss, reduce the risk of fractures, and improve overall bone health. By combining lifestyle modifications, appropriate medications if necessary, and regular follow-ups with healthcare professionals, individuals with osteopenia can take important steps towards maintaining strong and healthy bones throughout their lives.

Other Bone–Related Conditions and Treatments

Apart from osteoporosis and osteopenia, there are other bone-related conditions that can affect individuals, each with its own set of challenges and treatment options. Let's explore some of these conditions and the solutions available for managing them:

1. Paget's Disease of Bone:
Paget's disease is a chronic condition that disrupts the normal bone remodeling process, leading to the formation of weaker and enlarged bones. It can affect a single bone or multiple bones in the body and is more common in older individuals. Symptoms may include bone pain, deformities, and an increased risk of fractures.

Treatment: Treatment for Paget's disease may involve medications to regulate bone remodeling, reduce bone pain, and improve bone density. In some cases, surgery might be necessary to correct bone deformities or stabilize weakened bones.

2. Bone Tumors:

Bone tumors can be either benign (non-cancerous) or malignant (cancerous). Benign bone tumors do not spread to other parts of the body and are usually not life-threatening. Malignant bone tumors, on the other hand, require prompt and aggressive treatment.

Treatment: Treatment for bone tumors depends on their type, location, and whether they are benign or malignant. Options may include surgery to remove the tumor, chemotherapy, radiation therapy, and targeted therapies for cancerous tumors.

3. Osteogenesis Imperfecta (OI):

OI, also known as brittle bone disease, is a genetic disorder characterized by fragile bones that break easily, often with little or no apparent cause. It is caused by a deficiency in collagen, a protein crucial for bone strength.

Treatment: While there is no cure for OI, management focuses on preventing fractures and maximizing bone health. This may involve physical therapy, assistive devices to improve mobility, and medications to increase bone density and reduce fracture risk.

4. Fibrous Dysplasia:

Fibrous dysplasia is a rare bone disorder where fibrous tissue replaces normal bone, leading to weak and deformed bones. It can occur in a single bone (monostotic) or multiple bones (polyostotic).

Treatment: Treatment for fibrous dysplasia depends on the extent of the condition and the bones affected. In some cases, surgery may be necessary to stabilize the bone or correct deformities. Medications can also help manage symptoms and reduce bone pain.

5. Rickets and Osteomalacia:

Rickets and osteomalacia are conditions characterized by softening and weakening of the bones, primarily due to a deficiency of vitamin D, calcium, or phosphate.

Treatment: Treatment for rickets and osteomalacia involves addressing the underlying nutrient deficiencies. This may include vitamin D and calcium supplementation, along with dietary changes to ensure an adequate intake of these nutrients.

6. Bone Infections (Osteomyelitis):

Osteomyelitis is a bacterial or fungal infection of the bone that can be acute or chronic. It can occur due to open fractures, surgical procedures, or bloodstream infections.

Treatment: Treatment for osteomyelitis typically involves intravenous antibiotics to eliminate the infection. In severe cases, surgery may be necessary to remove infected bone tissue.

It is essential to consult a healthcare professional for accurate diagnosis and appropriate treatment for any bone-related condition. Early detection and proper management can significantly improve the quality of life for individuals with these conditions and reduce the risk of complications such as fractures and deformities. By combining medical interventions, lifestyle modifications, and preventive measures, individuals can take charge of their bone health and overall well-being.

Chapter 10: Building a Personalized Bone-Healthy Diet Plan

Maintaining strong and healthy bones is essential for overall well-being and quality of life. As we age, our bones become more susceptible to conditions like osteoporosis, which can lead to fractures and other bone-related issues. One effective way to support bone health is through a well-balanced and personalized diet plan that provides the necessary nutrients for bone strength. In this guide, we will explore the key components of a personalized bone-healthy diet plan.

1. Calcium-Rich Foods:

Calcium is a crucial mineral for bone health as it helps build and maintain bone density. Incorporate calcium-rich foods into your daily diet, such as dairy products like milk, yogurt, and cheese. If you are lactose intolerant or follow a plant-based diet, consider alternative sources of calcium such as fortified plant-based milks (soy, almond, etc.), tofu, leafy green vegetables (kale, broccoli, bok choy), and canned fish with edible bones (like sardines and salmon).

2. Vitamin D:

Vitamin D is vital for the absorption of calcium. It helps the body utilize calcium effectively and plays a significant role in bone health. Exposure to sunlight is one of the best natural sources of vitamin D. However, depending solely on sunlight might not be sufficient for everyone, especially in regions with limited sun exposure or during winter months. To ensure adequate vitamin D intake, include foods like fatty fish (salmon, mackerel, tuna), egg yolks, and fortified foods in your diet. You may also consider vitamin D supplements, but consult with a healthcare professional to determine the right dosage for you.

3. Magnesium:

Magnesium is another essential mineral for bone health, as it assists in converting vitamin D into its active form. Nuts, seeds, whole grains, legumes, leafy green vegetables, and seafood are excellent sources of magnesium that can be included in your diet plan.

4. Phosphorus:

Phosphorus is a mineral that works in conjunction with calcium to strengthen bones and teeth. Most people get enough phosphorus through their regular diet, as it is present in a wide range of foods, including dairy products, meat, poultry, fish, nuts, and whole grains.

5. Vitamin K:

Vitamin K is crucial for bone formation and remodeling. It helps regulate calcium levels in the body and contributes to bone density. Leafy green vegetables (kale, spinach, collard greens), broccoli, and Brussels sprouts are excellent sources of vitamin K.

6. Protein:

Protein is essential for bone health, as it provides the building blocks for bone tissue. Include adequate protein in your diet from sources such as lean meats, poultry, fish, beans, lentils, tofu, nuts, and seeds. A well-balanced protein intake also supports muscle health, which is essential for overall bone support.

7. Limit Caffeine and Alcohol:

Excessive consumption of caffeine and alcohol can interfere with calcium absorption and increase calcium excretion, potentially weakening bones. While moderate intake is generally safe, try to limit your consumption of caffeinated and alcoholic beverages to support optimal bone health.

8. Maintain a Healthy Weight and Exercise Regularly:

Maintaining a healthy weight through a balanced diet and regular exercise is crucial for bone health. Engage in weight-bearing exercises such as walking, jogging, dancing, and resistance training, as they help stimulate bone growth and improve bone density.

9. Consult with a Healthcare Professional:

Every individual is unique, and nutritional needs may vary depending on age, gender, medical conditions, and lifestyle factors

Assessing Your Nutritional Needs

Maintaining strong and healthy bones is crucial for overall well-being and preventing conditions like osteoporosis. A key component of bone health is a well-balanced diet that provides the necessary nutrients to support bone density and strength. Building a personalized bone-healthy diet plan begins with understanding your individual nutritional needs and making appropriate adjustments to your eating habits. Here are some essential steps to assess your nutritional needs and design a diet plan that promotes bone health.

1. Consult with a Healthcare Professional:
Before embarking on any significant dietary changes, it is essential to consult with a healthcare professional, such as a registered dietitian or a

doctor. They can assess your current bone health, identify any risk factors or deficiencies, and provide personalized guidance based on your medical history, lifestyle, and individual needs.

2. Evaluate Calcium Intake:

Calcium is a crucial mineral for bone health, as it contributes to bone structure and strength. Assess your daily calcium intake from dietary sources, such as dairy products, leafy greens (kale, broccoli, collard greens), fortified plant-based milk, and calcium-rich seafood (salmon, sardines). If your current intake is inadequate, your healthcare professional may recommend calcium supplements to meet your daily requirements.

3. Monitor Vitamin D Levels:

Vitamin D is essential for calcium absorption, making it a vital nutrient for bone health. Check your vitamin D levels through a blood test to determine if you have a deficiency. Sunlight is a natural source of vitamin D, but dietary sources like fatty fish (salmon, mackerel), fortified foods (cereals, orange juice), and supplements may be necessary, especially in regions with limited sunlight exposure.

4. Assess Magnesium and Vitamin K Intake:

Magnesium and vitamin K are two lesser-known but equally important nutrients for bone health. Magnesium aids in converting vitamin D into its active form, while vitamin K helps regulate calcium metabolism and promotes bone formation. Foods like nuts, seeds, whole grains, dark leafy greens, and fermented soy products are excellent sources of these nutrients.

5. Protein and Bone Health:

Protein is essential for maintaining bone mass and strength. Assess your protein intake to ensure it meets your individual needs. Include a variety of protein sources, such as lean meats, poultry, fish, dairy products, legumes, and plant-based alternatives like tofu and tempeh, to optimize bone health.

6. Watch Sodium and Caffeine Intake:

High sodium intake can lead to calcium excretion, potentially weakening bones. Similarly, excessive caffeine consumption can interfere with calcium absorption. Be mindful of your sodium and caffeine intake and try to limit processed foods and drinks high in caffeine.

7. Consider Other Bone-Supporting Nutrients:
Phosphorus, potassium, and various vitamins (A, C, and B) also play essential roles in bone health. A well-balanced diet that includes a variety of fruits, vegetables, whole grains, and lean protein sources can help ensure you get an adequate supply of these nutrients.

Designing a personalized bone-healthy diet plan begins with a comprehensive assessment of your nutritional needs. Partner with a healthcare professional to evaluate your calcium, vitamin D, magnesium, and vitamin K levels. Consider your protein, sodium, and caffeine intake, and aim for a well-rounded diet that incorporates a variety of bone-supporting nutrients. By making informed dietary choices and nurturing your bone health, you can take proactive steps towards maintaining strong and resilient bones throughout your life.

Creating Balanced Meals

A bone-healthy diet plan is not just about individual nutrients; it's also about how you combine them to create balanced meals that support optimal bone health. Designing meals that are rich in bone-supporting nutrients while being enjoyable and sustainable is essential for long-term success. Here are some guidelines for creating balanced meals that promote strong and healthy bones:

1. Prioritize Calcium-Rich Foods:
Calcium is a cornerstone of bone health, so make sure to incorporate calcium-rich foods into your meals. Include dairy products like milk, yogurt, and cheese if you are not lactose intolerant or prefer plant-based options, choose fortified plant-based milk, such as almond, soy, or oat milk. Additionally, load up on leafy greens like broccoli, kale, and collard greens, as well as calcium-fortified foods like tofu and orange juice.

2. Combine Calcium and Vitamin D:

Vitamin D enhances calcium absorption, making it essential to pair these two nutrients in your meals. Enjoy calcium-rich foods with vitamin D sources such as fatty fish (salmon, mackerel), egg yolks, and fortified foods. Consider having a vitamin D-rich snack like yogurt topped with berries, which provides both nutrients.

3. Include Lean Proteins:

Protein is essential for maintaining bone mass and strength. Opt for lean protein sources like skinless poultry, fish, beans, lentils, and tofu. Mix and match these proteins in salads, stir-fries, or sandwiches to add variety and flavor to your meals.

4. Don't Forget Magnesium and Vitamin K:

Incorporate foods rich in magnesium and vitamin K to complement your calcium intake. Magnesium sources include nuts, seeds, whole grains, and leafy greens, while vitamin K can be found in dark leafy greens like spinach and Swiss chard, as well as fermented soy products like natto.

5. Embrace Fruits and Vegetables:

Fruits and vegetables are essential for overall health and bone health as well. They provide a range of nutrients, including potassium, vitamin C, and antioxidants that contribute to bone health. Aim for a colorful plate filled with a variety of fruits and vegetables to maximize the nutritional benefits.

6. Add Healthy Fats:

Healthy fats play a role in overall health and can complement your bone-healthy diet. Incorporate sources of unsaturated fats like avocados, olive oil, and nuts into your meals to promote satiety and enhance nutrient absorption.

7. Limit Sodium and Caffeine:

High sodium intake can lead to calcium loss, while excessive caffeine can interfere with calcium absorption. Be mindful of your sodium intake and opt for lower-sodium alternatives. Limit caffeine consumption from sources like coffee, tea, and energy drinks and balance it with calcium-rich foods.

8. Hydrate with Water:

Proper hydration is essential for overall health and can also benefit bone health. Make water your primary beverage of choice, as it aids in nutrient absorption and supports bodily functions.

Building a personalized bone-healthy diet plan involves creating balanced meals that supply the necessary nutrients to support bone health. Prioritize calcium-rich foods, combine them with vitamin D sources, and include a variety of lean proteins, fruits, and vegetables. Don't forget about magnesium and vitamin K, and add healthy fats while limiting sodium and caffeine intake. By embracing a diverse and well-balanced diet, you can nourish your bones and pave the way for a lifetime of strong and healthy skeletal support. Remember to consult with a healthcare professional or a registered dietitian to ensure your personalized diet plan meets your unique nutritional needs and lifestyle.

Sample Meal Plans for Bone Health

Maintaining strong and healthy bones is essential for overall well-being, especially as we age. A bone-healthy diet plays a crucial role in providing the necessary nutrients to support bone density and prevent conditions like osteoporosis. This article will guide you through the process of creating a personalized bone-healthy diet plan and provide sample meal plans to get you started on the right track.

1. Understanding Bone-Boosting Nutrients:

Before diving into the meal plans, it's essential to understand the nutrients that are particularly beneficial for bone health:

a. Calcium: Calcium is the primary mineral responsible for building and maintaining strong bones. Good sources of calcium include dairy products (milk, yogurt, and cheese), leafy green vegetables (kale, broccoli, bok choy), and fortified plant-based milk.

b. Vitamin D: Vitamin D is essential for calcium absorption. Exposure to sunlight is one of the best ways to get vitamin D, but you can also find it in fatty fish (salmon, mackerel), egg yolks, and fortified foods.

c. Magnesium: Magnesium works in tandem with calcium to support bone health. Nuts, seeds, whole grains, and leafy greens are excellent sources of magnesium.

d. Vitamin K: Vitamin K helps regulate calcium and promote bone mineralization. Green leafy vegetables (spinach, collard greens) and cruciferous vegetables (broccoli, Brussels sprouts) are rich in vitamin K.

e. Protein: Adequate protein intake is necessary for maintaining bone mass. Sources of protein include lean meats, poultry, fish, beans, lentils, and tofu.

2. Creating a Personalized Bone-Healthy Diet Plan:

Every individual has unique dietary needs, so it's crucial to personalize your bone-healthy diet plan based on factors such as age, gender, lifestyle, and any specific dietary restrictions or health conditions. Consult with a registered dietitian or healthcare professional to tailor a plan to your specific needs. However, the following sample meal plans can serve as a general guide:

Sample Meal Plan 1: Balanced Diet

- Breakfast:
  - Greek yogurt with sliced strawberries and a sprinkle of almonds.
  - Whole-grain toast with avocado spread.

- Snack:
  - Carrot sticks with hummus.

- Lunch:

- Grilled chicken salad with mixed greens, cherry tomatoes, cucumber, and a drizzle of olive oil and lemon dressing.
  - Quinoa and vegetable soup.

- Snack:

  - A small handful of mixed nuts.

- Dinner:

  - Baked salmon with lemon and dill.
  - Steamed broccoli and sautéed kale.
  - Brown rice.

- Dessert (optional):

  - A serving of frozen yogurt with a handful of blueberries.

Sample Meal Plan 2: Plant-Based Diet

- Breakfast:

  - Smoothie with spinach, banana, almond milk, chia seeds, and a scoop of plant-based protein powder.

- Snack:

- Sliced cucumber with tahini dip.

- Lunch:

- Chickpea and vegetable stir-fry with tofu.

- Quinoa salad with kale, cherry tomatoes, and a lemon-tahini dressing.

- Snack:

- Dried apricots and pumpkin seeds.

- Dinner:

- Baked sweet potato with black bean and avocado salsa.

- Grilled asparagus.

- Dessert (optional):

- Chia seed pudding with coconut milk and topped with fresh berries.

3. General Tips for a Bone-Healthy Diet:

- Limit processed foods and excessive salt intake, as they may lead to calcium loss.

- Avoid sugary sodas and excessive caffeine, which may interfere with calcium absorption.
- Engage in regular weight-bearing exercises, as they promote bone strength.

These sample meal plans are just a starting point. Customize them to fit your tastes and preferences while ensuring they include a variety of bone-boosting nutrients. For optimal bone health, consistency is key, so make this bone-healthy diet plan a lifestyle choice to reap long-term benefits for your bones and overall well-being.

Conclusion

building a personalized bone-healthy diet plan is a proactive and essential step towards maintaining strong and healthy bones throughout life. By focusing on nutrient-rich foods and incorporating a variety of bone-boosting nutrients like calcium, vitamin D, magnesium, vitamin K, and protein, you can support bone density and reduce the risk of bone-related conditions like osteoporosis.

The sample meal plans provided are just examples, and it's crucial to tailor your diet based on your individual needs, preferences, and health status. Consulting with a registered dietitian or healthcare professional can help create a plan that addresses your specific requirements and ensures you are getting the right balance of nutrients.

In addition to following a bone-healthy diet, remember that a healthy lifestyle also includes regular physical activity, especially weight-bearing exercises, which further

Furthermore, a bone-healthy diet not only benefits bone health but also contributes to overall wellness. Many of the foods rich in bone-boosting nutrients are also packed with other essential vitamins and minerals that support various bodily functions, such as immune health, cardiovascular health, and digestive health.

It's essential to maintain consistency in adhering to your bone-healthy diet plan. While immediate results may not be visible, long-term dedication to a nutrient-rich diet can yield substantial benefits, especially as you age. Building strong bones during your younger years sets the foundation for a healthier future, reducing the risk of fractures and bone-related problems as you get older.

Remember that every stage of life has unique nutritional requirements. Whether you are a child, teenager, adult, or senior, your bone-healthy diet plan should evolve accordingly. Regularly review your dietary choices and adjust them to meet your changing needs.

As you embark on your bone health journey, be patient and kind to yourself. Making lifestyle changes, including dietary modifications, can be challenging, but small, sustainable steps can lead to significant improvements over time. Embrace the process and celebrate your progress along the way.

Incorporate a wide variety of bone-boosting foods into your daily meals, and consider experimenting with new recipes and flavors to keep your diet exciting and enjoyable. Engage with others who share similar health goals, as a support system can make the journey more manageable and motivating.

a bone-healthy diet plan is an investment in your long-term well-being. By prioritizing nutrient-dense foods, staying physically active, and adopting a holistic approach to health, you can nurture your bones and pave the way for a vibrant and active life. Remember, it's never too late to start taking care of your bones, so begin your bone-healthy journey today and savor the benefits of stronger, healthier bones fAbuildingalthy diet plan is an investment in your long-term well-being. By prioritizing nutrient-dense foods, staying physically active, and adopting a holistic approach to health, you can nurture your bones and pave the way for a vibrant and active life. Remember, it's never too late to start taking care of your bones, so begin your bone-healthy journey today and savor the benefits of stronger, healthier bones for years to come.building